FOREWORD BY **T. COLIN CAMPBELL, PhD**
AND **CALDWELL B. ESSELSTYN JR., MD**

THE PLANT-BASED WAY TO HEALTH

D0011178

FORKS OVER KNIVES

EDITED BY GENE STONE

WITH CONTRIBUTIONS BY **PAM POPPER, ND, MICAELA COOK,**
ELISE MURPHY, AND MEGHAN MURPHY

THE EXPERIMENT

NEW YORK

DEDICATED TO

*T. Colin Campbell, PhD, Caldwell B. Esselstyn, Jr., MD,
and all the researchers who have committed their lives to improving
our understanding of the relationship between food and health.*

The Experiment, LLC
260 Fifth Avenue
New York, NY 10001–6408
www.theexperimentpublishing.com

Many of the designations used by manufacturers and sellers to distinguish their products are claimed as trademarks. Where those designations appear in this book and The Experiment was aware of a trademark claim, the designations have been capitalized.

The Experiment's books are available at special discounts when purchased in bulk for premiums and sales promotions as well as for fundraising or educational use. For details, contact us at info@theexperimentpublishing.com.

The statements expressed in this book are not meant to be a substitute for professional medical advice. Readers should seek their own professional counsel for any medical condition or before starting or altering any exercise or dietary plan.

Library of Congress Control Number: 2011929967
ISBN 978-1-61519-045-4
Ebook ISBN 978-1-61519-146-8

Cover design by Kathy Kikkert
Cover photographs by Bigstock.com
Text design by Pauline Neuwirth, Neuwirth & Associates, Inc.

Manufactured in the United States of America
Distributed by Workman Publishing Company, Inc.
Distributed simultaneously in Canada by Thomas Allen & Son Limited

First published June 2011
10 9 8

CONTENTS

FOREWORD

By T. Colin Campbell, PhD, and Caldwell B. Esselstyn, Jr., MD

Leave your drugs in the chemist's pot
if you can cure the patient with food.
—HIPPOCRATES

For more than 2,800 years, the concept of eating plants in their whole-food form has struggled to be heard and adopted as a way of life. Although it is usually defended on ideological grounds, recent evidence now proves that this diet produces powerful personal health benefits as well. In fact, eating a plant-based diet has become an urgent matter from several perspectives: Not only can personal health be improved but also health care costs can be dramatically reduced, and various forms of violence to our environment and to other sentient beings can be minimized.

Because this diet has so much to offer, we believe that the means must be found to share this information with as many people as possible, people of all persuasions and backgrounds, regardless of age, gender, ethnicity, and geographic location. And one of the best ways to accomplish this is through sharing personal experiences and imagery, as in the film *Forks Over Knives*.

Forks Over Knives is both a journey and a saga. The journey demonstrates how rapidly health can be restored without drugs, medications, and surgical procedures. The saga presents the individual tales of those whose profound lifestyle changes have halted and even reversed serious diseases.

Our nation's economic stability has been crumbling because of the burst bubbles in technology and housing. This burden has been compounded by spiraling health costs, with no end in sight. Yet, as a nation we are sicker and fatter than we have ever been. The epidemics of obesity and diabetes, especially in the young, forecasts an economically unsustainable public health challenge and the gloomy prophecy that today's children may not outlive their parents.

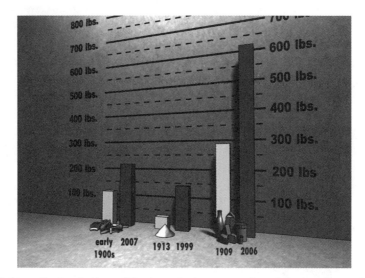

Figure 1: Near the beginning of the twentieth century, Americans each ate about 120 pounds of meat yearly; as of 2007, we ate about 222 pounds. In 1913, we consumed about 40 pounds of processed sugar each; by 1999, that number had risen to 147 pounds. And, in 1909, Americans downed 294 pounds of dairy products apiece—by 2006, that figure had more than doubled to 605 pounds per person.

The central protagonist of this dark scenario is the food industry and its profit demands. With billions of advertising and marketing dollars, it annually cajoles and entices us with its dairy, meat, fish, poultry, and eggs, as well as products laden with sugar, salt, and fat. This ceaseless assault achieves its goal of convincing a vulnerable and unprotected public to ingest food that will make them fat and sick: Obesity, hypertension, diabetes, heart disease, strokes, cancer, rheumatoid arthritis, multiple sclerosis, lupus, gallstones, diverticulitis, osteoporosis, allergies, and asthma are but a few of the diseases of Western nutrition.

Who will protect the public? Not our government: The U.S. Department of Agriculture is the voice of our food industry. Every five years it constructs nutrition guidelines for the public touting food that will guarantee ill health for millions. Not the American Dietetic Association, which is controlled by food corporations. Not the insurance industry, which profits by selling plans to the sick. Not the pharmaceutical industry, which pockets billions annually from chronic illnesses. Not hospitals, whose livelihood depends on our diseases. Not the medical profession, in which doctors and nurses receive virtually no training in nutrition or behavioral modification, and are handsomely rewarded for administrating drugs and employing technical expertise. And, finally, not our medical research funding institutions: Too often they focus on biological details, such as individual nutrients, that can be exploited commercially for profit.

The primary focus of *Forks Over Knives* is whole-foods, plant-based nutrition. The public needs new avenues to understand this message, and that is why this film is so important. A seismic revolution in health will not come from a pill, procedure, or operation. It will occur only when the public is endowed with nutritional literacy, the kind of knowledge portrayed in *Forks Over Knives* and highlighted by this book.

Once you see the movie, we hope you will make the transition to this dietary lifestyle. It may loom like a challenge. But it's only because so many of us have become addicted to diets high in fat, salt, and sugar that the adventure of eating foods that contain few of these ingredients seems so difficult. It isn't. We know from both anecdotal experience and from the scientific literature that such addictions can be resolved in a matter of weeks.

So, stick with it, eat well, and you will soon discover a whole new universe of gustatory pleasure, savoring new tastes never before recognized. Please try some of the recipes in this book to help you make this transition. You will find these foods taste superb and are reasonably easy to prepare. It is with this thought in mind that we entrust to you this idea and these recipes to set you on your path. Bon appétit!

PART ONE

The Plant-Based World of

FORKS OVER KNIVES

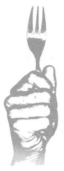

GOOD FOR
YOUR HEALTH

One quarter of what you eat keeps you alive. The other three
quarters keep your doctor alive.
—EGYPTIAN PROVERB

Good health. Throughout recorded history, health has been one of our most common preoccupations and most popular areas of research. In fact, the study of medicine predates written history. In 1991, the discovery of a 5,000-year-old mummified body in Northern Italy revealed that prehistoric societies had greater medical knowledge than once thought: The man, now known as Otzi the Iceman, had among his possessions a fungus that scientists discovered can kill internal parasites—the first palpable evidence of early human pharmacology.

Going back further in time, we know that shamans and healers used various plants and herbs (as well as magical chants and prayers) as medication in the earliest societies on record; every culture had some form of medicinal wisdom, although almost all of that knowledge is lost to us today.

Today, if you Google the word *health* you'll see about 2 billion results— interest in health has probably never been greater than it is today. Health information is endemic in our culture: It's plastered on everything from cereal boxes to billboards, featured in magazine and newspaper articles, discussed on daytime talk shows and on prime-time news programs, and disseminated in costly newsletters and private seminars. Health-related books dominate the best-seller lists. Health-related products are sold everywhere, from drugstores to late-night infomercials.

You might think all this interest would result in good health for most people. It hasn't. Most Americans are sick. In the United States, one person is killed by heart disease every minute. Every day, 1,500 people die from cancer. Combined, these two diseases kill over one million people per year. The Centers for Disease Control estimate that seven out of ten deaths are from chronic diseases.

For Americans between the ages of 45 and 64, the rate of suffering from three or more chronic diseases jumped from 13 percent in 1996 to 22 percent in 2005. Overall, between 1996 and 2005, the number of Americans of all ages who suffer from three or more chronic diseases increased by 86 percent. And in the past decade alone, the incidence of diabetes has grown 90 percent.

On top of that, two thirds of adults are either overweight or obese, and obesity rates for children have doubled over the past thirty years. More than 24 million Americans suffer from diabetes, most cases of which are a result of the same poor diet that led to their obesity. And this number will only increase: An estimated 57 million Americans are experiencing "pre-diabetic" symptoms.

A growing number of people are becoming aware that lifestyle choices can have a powerful effect on their health, and paramount among those choices is nutrition. However, in spite of this knowledge, most people are still eating a health-destroying diet rich in fatty, salty, sugary junk and animal-based foods. Unfortunately, the link between diet and health is still not well understood by many doctors, who are not required to take courses on nutrition in school, and who therefore rely on pills and procedures to treat patients.

Furthermore, vested interests in the food and agriculture industries have spent millions of dollars each year on marketing that discourages people from associating bad health with bad food. The pharmaceutical industry, which promotes the use of drugs over food for maintaining health, retains 1,585 lobbyists, on whom it spends over $241 million per year.

But could the answer to our health problems be a relatively straightforward one? Could it be that the best way to promote health and to avoid disease isn't to take large quantities of medicines, or to rely on complicated medical procedures?

The answer is *yes*. The formula for good health may be as simple as this: Eating a whole-foods, plant-based diet. That's what the world of *Forks Over Knives* is all about, and it's a message that is resonating with audiences nationwide.

A PLANT-BASED DIET

A plant-based diet is a very simple one. It consists of avoiding anything that came from a source that ever had a face or a mother. In other words, avoiding all meat (including fish), dairy, and eggs.

What you do eat are the very best foods that Mother Nature offers: grains, fruits, vegetables, and legumes. Often relegated to side dishes by a meat-devouring American public, these foods actually create the best-tasting and most nutritious meals possible.

A healthy, plant-based diet is also composed of whole foods. That means avoiding refined foods, such as olive oil and white bread, and staying away from artificial foods with chemical additives. In other words, a plant-based diet is centered on foods that come from whole, unrefined plants. As Dr. John McDougall (page 52) says, "There is a right diet for humans," and it is based on one key principle: Eat plants. (It isn't just Dr. McDougall who believes this. Another famous thinker, Charles Darwin, said, "The normal food of man is vegetable.")

Here are the key principles of the plant-based, whole-foods, *Forks Over Knives* diet:

▶ **EAT PLANTS—THE MORE INTACT, THE BETTER.** And not just any plants—eat whole, minimally refined fruit, vegetables, grains, and legumes. The closer you can get to the plant as it exists in nature, the better. Natural, plant-based foods provide all the essential nutrients needed for a well-balanced and healthy diet, as there are no nutrients found in animal-based foods that are not abundantly available in plant foods (with the exception of vitamin B_{12}; see below).

This means that a diet of potato chips, pretzels, dairy-free pastries, and low-calorie soda may technically be a plant-based diet, but it is not a healthy plant-based diet.

A well-structured, plant-based diet will meet all your nutritional needs—for calories, protein, vitamins, and minerals—without calorie counting, portion control, or measuring. It's the easiest way to eat!

▶ **AVOID OVERLY PROCESSED FOODS.** These are foods that include, among other items, bleached flour, refined sugars, and extracted oils. White flours, sugars, and most oils do come from plants, but they have been stripped of most of the nutritional properties they once had. And although some nutritionists recommend olive oil, why cook with the most concentrated form of fat on the planet when you can choose from many other liquids? Olives are a wonderful food, but olive oil can be problematic.

The reason? Oil is 100 percent pure fat. This means that, in the case of olive oil for instance, the manufacturers have taken whole olives, squeezed out and chemically extracted the good parts (the healthy fiber, vitamins, and minerals), and left you with little more than a concentrated dose of calories. Olive oil contains close to 4,100 calories per 16 ounces!

▶ **AVOID PRESERVATIVES AND ADDITIVES.** This is a no-brainer. Why load up your diet with anything artificial when you can be eating whole foods that don't need additives to make them taste so great?

▶ **ELIMINATE DAIRY.** Casein, the primary protein in cow's milk, may well be one of the most potent chemical carcinogens ever identified (to learn more, read Colin Campbell's *The China Study*; see page 20). Dairy products increase the risk for chronic diseases, and cow's milk in particular has been linked to an increased risk for cancer, juvenile diabetes, multiple sclerosis, and many other conditions.

Humans have no nutritional need for cow's milk. Cow's milk is designed to provide a baby calf with adequate nutrients to grow from 70 pounds to about 1,000 pounds in one year. And, it contains casomorphins, addictive compounds similar to morphine, to ensure that the calf will stay near its mother, safely nursing and growing. Casomorphins are addictive for humans as well, which can make giving up dairy a challenge.

▶ **DON'T WORRY ABOUT CARBOHYDRATES.** Nearly everyone has heard about low-carbohydrate diets—they have been fashionable for years. But they are not necessarily healthy. In fact, carbohydrates are the body's preferred energy source, so it's important to eat carbohydrate-rich foods.

It's also important to choose the right *types* of carbohydrate-rich foods. Mangoes, broccoli, and pastries are all high-carbohydrate foods, but mangoes and broccoli are obviously much better for you. If you eat cakes and cookies made with white flour and sugar, you'll experience rapid rises in blood-sugar levels, increased insulin response, and weight gain. If you eat whole-plant foods like fruits, whole grains, and vegetables, you'll thrive on a high-carbohydrate diet. As an added bonus, these foods are high in fiber, which provides a feeling of fullness. Eating high-fiber foods almost always reduces the overall number of calories consumed, which assists with weight loss.

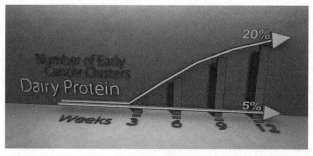

Figure 2a

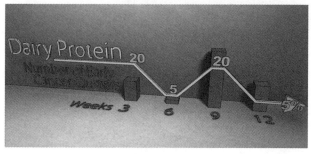

Figure 2b

Figure 2a: To test his theory about dairy, Dr. Colin Campbell fed two groups of rats diets with different amounts of casein, the main protein in dairy products. After 12 weeks, all of the rats eating a diet of 20 percent casein had a greatly increased level of early cancer tumor growth, while rats eating a 5 percent diet showed no evidence of cancer whatsoever.

Figure 2b: Dr. Campbell then switched the rats' diets back and forth—between 5 and 20 percent dairy protein. Whenever the rats were fed 20 percent protein, early liver tumor growth exploded; when the same rats were given 5 percent protein, tumor growth actually went down. In *Forks Over Knives*, Dr. Campbell says, "We learned that we could turn on and turn off cancer growth—just by adjusting the level of intake of that protein."

▶ **DON'T WORRY ABOUT NOT GETTING ENOUGH PROTEIN.** One of the most common myths about a plant-based diet is that you won't get enough protein. This is simply untrue. Plant foods contain plenty of protein, and a whole-foods, plant-based diet provides an appropriate level of total dietary protein—around 10 percent of total calories. That proportion exceeds the level required for most people.

One useful principle to keep in mind: It is impossible to structure a diet that provides enough calories but does not provide enough protein. The word for malnutrition caused by a protein deficiency isn't even known to the vast majority of Americans. (It's *kwashiorkor!*)

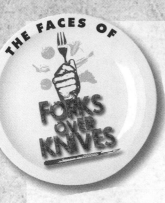

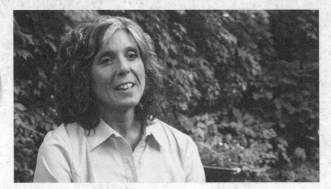

Pam Popper, ND

NATUROPATH PAM POPPER is the executive director of the Wellness Forum, which offers educational programs to help individuals improve their health, help employers reduce their health-care costs, and help health-care professionals enhance their patients' diet and lifestyle. She also works with the Physicians Committee for Responsible Medicine, and with Whole Foods Market, teaching the supermarket chain's employees to improve their health using plant-based nutrition. Additionally, she is a featured lecturer in Colin Campbell's online courses through eCornell. Her most recent book is *Solving America's Healthcare Crisis*.

Pam, who was born in Ohio in 1956, didn't expect to pursue a career in health. Until she was twenty-eight, she was a salesperson who smoked four packs of cigarettes daily and, until she was thirty-eight, ate whatever foods she felt like eating. "I was nutritionally unconscious," she says. Then, eighteen years ago, a friend gave her a book by Dr. John McDougall. "I thought I was a smart person, I thought I knew a lot, but I didn't know about this."

She liked the book and decided to read more about the relationship between diet and health. "This is it," she thought. "This is what I want to be when I grow up." Today, she operates a nutrition-based private practice out of her office in Ohio and has clients all over the world.

"For me, the big change is that, before, my job was just a job. Now, I love what I do. People in the medical field usually have unhappy days, but I almost always see people get better."

Critics of a plant-based diet, says Pam, contend that people won't change what they eat. "But I find that the issue is that most patients are not making informed choices; doctors simply tell them, for example, that their cholesterol is too high and that they should go on statins. They don't offer a choice.

We tell patients that they can indeed go on statins, in which case they will experience negative side effects, or they can change their diet, which won't have side effects, won't cost additional money, and will protect them from a stroke or heart attack. Most people aren't being given the information this way. If they were, they'd be more likely to change.

"The other issue critics bring up is that people won't stick with a new diet. But I see people doing it all the time. When you make big changes in your diet, your health improves quickly. Our clients tell us that they no longer want cheese, cookies, and cakes anymore. Going back to bad foods means going back to taking medications and even spending time in the hospital. They'd rather be healthy.

"A plant-based diet may seem restrictive when you first hear about it, but actually it lets you do whatever you want to do with the maximum amount of energy for all the years that you are on this planet. It's not what's being taken away. It's what you're getting."

▶ **DON'T WORRY ABOUT OMEGA-3 FATTY ACIDS.** There are two essential fatty acids, meaning you must consume them in foods—omega-3 and omega-6. Humans have historically consumed a diet with a ratio of omega-3 to omega-6 fatty acids ranging from 1:1 to 1:4. In recent years, as consumption of animal foods and polyunsaturated vegetable oils (in processed foods) has increased, this ratio has changed dramatically: The range is now about 1:25 to 1:30. As a result, many health-care professionals are suggesting that people take omega-3 supplements such as fish oil or increase their consumption of fish to correct this imbalance. But supplements cause side effects, and fish oil is not a great option because it contains cholesterol, saturated fat, and often mercury and other toxins. (There are also negative ecological implications of eating fish—see page 38). The better option is to eat a well-structured, plant-based diet, which reduces the consumption of omega-6 fatty acids and negates the need to increase your intake of omega-3 fatty acids.

▶ **CONSIDER A VITAMIN B$_{12}$ SUPPLEMENT.** Vitamin B$_{12}$ is a crucial vitamin, necessary for the proper functioning of the brain and the nervous system. Most people get their vitamin B$_{12}$ from eating meat or other animal-based foods. But meat is not the initial source of the B$_{12}$: it actually comes from the bacteria in the soil in which plants grow—plants that are then eaten by the animals.

Soil is often rich in B$_{12}$, and that's how plant-eaters have always obtained most of their vitamin B$_{12}$—through the dirt that clings to the vegetables that come directly from the rich soil. However, today, food is so highly sanitized that all of this dirt is gone by the time we eat it.

People require very little B$_{12}$: The recommended daily allowance ranges from 0.4 to 2.8 micrograms. And the body stores 2 to 5 milligrams in adults—three orders of magnitude more than is needed each day—and those stores can last for several years.

The solution? Take a supplement for insurance. Check with a qualified health professional concerning appropriate dosage.

DIET-RELATED DISEASES

Most people tend to think that diseases such as cancer and coronary artery disease are the result of bad luck or bad genes. These conditions are considered incurable by many health-care professionals, since the drugs and surgeries commonly prescribed for them only treat symptoms. The truth is, smart choices at the grocery store and in the kitchen can prevent heart disease, stroke, diabetes, and many other conditions, and in many instances can stop or reverse them.

This section is only a summary of the relationship between serious illness and diet. For more information on the subject, see the Bookshelf (page 199).

Heart Disease

The term "heart disease" is misleading, implying that your heart muscle is prone to catching ailments like the flu or the common cold—as if heart disease is something that just happens to you. Many people blame high blood pressure or elevated cholesterol on non-lifestyle factors such as family history. "My grandparents had high blood pressure," they'll say, "so there's nothing I can do about it except to take medication." But, although genetics may play a role in your disease, your grandparents may well have had high blood pressure because they ate poorly.

Here's a frightening fact: The National Heart, Lung, and Blood Institute recently released a report based on the ten-year findings of their Cardiovascular Health Study, concluding that nearly all males over age sixty-five and females over seventy who have grown up eating a traditional, meat-based Western diet are already suffering from some form of heart disease.

In most cases, the root of coronary artery disease is plaque, a greasy, fatty deposit that builds up in arteries throughout our bodies. Healthy arteries are strong and elastic, and lined with a smooth, Teflon-like substance called endothelial tissue. Over time, as people ingest dietary fat and cholesterol, the endothelial cells become "sticky" and plaque begins accumulating. Plaque can also narrow the arterial passageways through which our blood delivers vital oxygen and nutrients to our body, which results in hypertension and, by closing off arteries, can cause cardiac arrest. Plaques can also rupture, spilling their toxic contents into the bloodstream, which activates platelets that try to control the damage by clotting. The resulting blockage can deprive the heart muscle of oxygen, causing a heart attack or even sudden death.

Although some modern medicines, such as nitroglycerin, help the heart receive more blood by chemically dilating the arteries, these address only a symptom of the real problem. Wider arteries simply mean more room for plaque to accumulate in later. Imagine commuting to work every day with

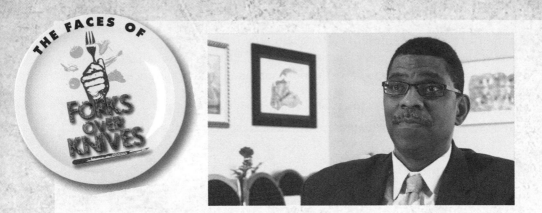

Terry Mason, MD

DR. TERRY MASON is the chief medical officer of the Cook County Health and Hospitals System in Illinois. He works with three hospitals; sixteen ambulatory clinics, some of which treat outpatients for HIV/AIDS and sexually transmitted diseases; a public health department; the local juvenile detention center; and the Cook County jail.

Terry grew up and was educated in and around Chicago. He then attended college at Loyola University and medical school at the University of Illinois and performed his residency in urology at Michael Reese Hospital. A board-certified urologist, Terry practiced medicine for twenty-five years before being named commissioner of the Chicago Department of Public Health in 2005. During his tenure there, he focused on fighting chronic disease by promoting healthier lifestyles.

Terry is also an inspirational speaker on the topic of building healthy communities. He hosts a radio talk show, *Doctor in the House*, and he is a frequent guest on national television and radio programs.

Terry took an unusual route to arrive at his current 98 percent plant-based philosophy (now and then he may eat an egg white or two). As a urologist, he found himself dealing with patients who had many challenging medical issues, particularly his specialty, erectile dysfunction.

"There was a strong link between men who had erection problems and men who had heart disease, something we discussed at a joint meeting of cardiologists and urologists at the National Medical Association convention to help us understand the link between the pathology for cardiovascular disease and that of erectile dysfunction.

"Soon, we found that this strong relationship was due to damage to the endothelial cells. The endothelium is the thin layer of cells that line the interior surface of blood vessels. Now, the penis has more endothelial cells per unit volume than any other organ in the body. So anything that would affect endothelial cell function would also pose a problem in the penis.

"As we also looked at the American diet, we found a strong correlation between damage to these endothelial cells and a meat-based, high-fat, high-calorie, and low-to-no exercise lifestyle. This lifestyle had a negative effect on both the penis and the heart.

"We are losing a million people a year to heart disease and cancer, and this is because of three things: smoking, the failure to exercise, and our poor diet. We need to address all three, and the right way to change that last issue is by adopting a plant-based diet. But we are going to have to take some radical steps to do so. When you adopt a public-health approach, you have to change society's basic structures in a way that will make it easier for people to do the right things and harder for them to do the wrong ones. I would put whatever resources are required into a government-led campaign to make fruits and veggies cheaper and more widely available and teach people how to prepare them.

"We are in a state of emergency! We can't continue to do what we are doing and expect different results. That's called insanity."

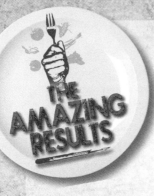

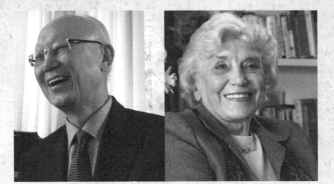

Anthony and Evelyn

FORKS OVER KNIVES chronicles many personal stories, including those of several people whose lives have been saved by switching to a whole-foods, plant-based diet—even after a lifetime of illness.

Among them are Anthony Yen and Evelyn Oswick. Anthony and Evelyn had each suffered multiple severe coronary events (heart attacks and bypass surgeries) and many years of chronic chest pain. Both had spent their lives making poor food choices, and the best options that their doctors had to offer them were merely palliative.

Evelyn recounts a conversation she had with her former cardiologist after her second heart attack: "I said, 'You mean that what you want me to do is buy a rocking chair and just sit there and rock away and wait?' And he just looked at me and said, 'Yes, that's just exactly what I'm saying.'"

Demographically speaking, Anthony started out with every advantage to protect him against heart disease. Born in China more than seventy years ago, he grew up eating what he calls a typical Chinese diet. Family meals centered on vegetables, rice, and soup, with only small servings of meat used as a seasoning, rather than the large portions served in the United States as a main course.

However, after moving to the United States as a young man and becoming a successful entrepreneur, Anthony started eating the typical Western diet, which emphasizes hamburgers, cheeseburgers, and pizza over whole, plant-based foods. Soon he was gaining weight, and he kept gaining weight in the years that followed. Anthony did a great deal of entertaining for business, and that meant countless fancy dinners featuring oysters, roast beef, steak, and shrimp.

All this indulgence lead to angina (chest pain) and a trip to the doctor's office, which was followed by a cardiogram, an angiogram, the diagnosis of a severe artery blockage, and finally, open-heart surgery with five bypasses—all this at the age of 55.

The net result of Anthony's surgery was more chest pain a week later. Fortunately, a cardiac specialist referred him to Dr. Caldwell Esselstyn, who soon had Anthony eating a whole-foods, plant-based diet.

Evelyn, also in her seventies, was a lover of doughnuts, desserts, chocolate, and thick sauces. She was first alerted to her own heart disease by a heart attack she suffered while pedaling on a stationary bike during a routine physical. Soon she was undergoing triple-bypass surgery.

Symptom-free before the surgery, Evelyn managed to get through another five years on her heart-killing diet before enduring a second cardiac incident. This time, bypass surgery wasn't recommended. Instead, she received the quiet suggestion that she while away her few remaining days on earth. Lucky for Evelyn, in what seemed like an afterthought her doctor mentioned that another physician, Dr. Esselstyn, was starting a new diet program for the heart and suggested she try it.

Evelyn's initial conversation with Dr. Esselstyn was short. He explained the foods she could and could not eat, and she made her decision.

"I'd rather die than be on your diet," she blurted.

"Okay, if that's the way you feel," Dr. Esselstyn replied.

But Evelyn soon decided that what she really felt was a desire to save her own life.

Both Evelyn and Anthony continued treatment under Dr. Esselstyn, who devoted a great deal of time to both of his new patients, explaining why they were going on this type of diet and listening for hours as they talked about their lives and their medical histories.

Like the overwhelming majority of Dr. Esselstyn's patients, Anthony and Evelyn successfully reversed their advanced-stage heart disease. In fact, not only have they survived far longer than their cardiologists had predicted, they are still living after what Dr. Esselstyn sometimes likes to call the heart-patient "warranty period" (25 years or 25,000 miles). Most important, today both Evelyn and Anthony are enjoying active lives full of friends, family, and meaningful work.

a leaking tire. You can pump air into the tire every morning, but wouldn't it make more sense to stop the leak? It's just going to become worse and worse until the day your tire blows out on the highway.

The same goes for our bodies. How do we fix our own leaky tire—that is, the buildup of dangerous plaque in our blood? The answer is simple: Avoid animal-based foods.

Animal-based foods are full of fat and cholesterol and leave us marinating in the very worst building blocks for heart disease. These foods contribute to the buildup of plaque along the sixty thousand miles of veins, arteries, and capillaries through which your blood must travel freely to keep you alive.

Plant-based foods, on the other hand, don't promote the accumulation of plaque and contain nutrients that can actually improve the health of your arteries and reverse the progression of heart disease.

Why? First and foremost, a healthful plant-based diet minimizes fat and cholesterol—the key components of artery-clogging plaque. With these dangerous plaque building blocks no longer inundating arteries after every meal, the body's natural healing processes are able to stabilize the plaque that has already built up, reducing cholesterol and allowing blood passageways to relax naturally.

Further evidence comes from Colin Campbell's China Study, a thirty-year investigation of the health and nutritional habits of 6,500 Chinese in sixty-five rural villages. After compiling their data, the researchers concluded that American men were seventeen times more likely to die from heart disease than rural Chinese men. In certain pockets of China where plant-based diets were most common, researchers could not find a single person out of more than 100,000 who had died from heart disease. While the average American's total cholesterol level is well over 200, the levels of the participants in the China Study averaged between 81 and 135. Dr. Campbell ultimately concluded that people who maintain a whole-foods, plant-based diet can minimize or even reverse the development of chronic diseases.

Still more evidence: Dr. Caldwell Esselstyn's twenty-year study at the Cleveland Clinic, which he wrote about in his book *Prevent and Reverse Heart Disease*, showed that a plant-based, oil-free diet will not just prevent heart disease but can even reverse it. Says Dr. Esselstyn, "Plaque does not develop until the endothelium, or the lining of the arteries, is injured—and it is injured every time people eat meat, dairy, fish, and chicken. This cannot be emphasized enough."

Stroke

Plaque can build up over time in the blood passageways leading to the brain as well as the heart. Even a momentary clot can deprive the brain of vital oxygen, which can result in permanent impairment. Every year, 700,000 Americans suffer a stroke, and for more than one-quarter of these victims, it proves fatal.

A whole-foods, plant-based diet has been proven to substantially reduce the risk of stroke. In fact, according to the remarkable fifty-year Framingham Heart Study conducted by the National Heart, Lung, and Blood Institute, for every three additional servings of fruits and vegetables you eat per day, your risk of stroke is reduced by 22 percent.

The Leading Causes of Death . . .

THE TEN LEADING CAUSES of death in the United States in 2007 (and numbers of fatalities):

- Heart disease: 616,067
- Cancer: 562,875
- Stroke (cerebrovascular diseases): 135,952
- Chronic lower respiratory diseases: 127,924
- Accidents (unintentional injuries): 123,706
- Alzheimer's disease: 74,632
- Diabetes: 71,382
- Influenza and Pneumonia: 52,717
- Nephritis, nephrotic syndrome, and nephrosis: 46,448
- Septicemia: 34,828

There is much evidence showing that heart disease, cancer, diabetes, stroke, and Alzheimer's disease are nutritionally related, so it could well be said that the leading cause of death in the United States in 2007 was poor nutrition.

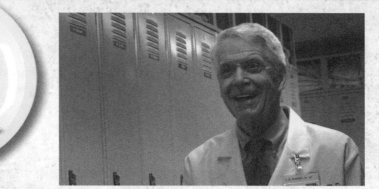

Caldwell B. Esselstyn Jr., MD

DR. CALDWELL B. Esselstyn Jr., known as Es, was educated at Yale and Case Western Reserve. (While at Yale, he won a gold medal at the 1956 Olympic Games as a member of the U.S. rowing team.) He trained as a surgeon at the Cleveland Clinic and at St. George's Hospital in London. In 1968, as an army surgeon in Vietnam, he was awarded the Bronze Star.

Es has been associated with the Cleveland Clinic since 1968, serving as the president of the staff, a member of its Board of Governors, chair of its Breast Cancer Task Force, and head of its division of thyroid and parathyroid surgery. In 1991, he served as president of the American Association of Endocrine Surgeons; in 2005, he was the first recipient of the Benjamin Spock Award for Compassion in Medicine; and in 2009, he received the Distinguished Alumnus Award from the Cleveland Clinic Alumni Association. Today Es runs the cardiovascular prevention and reversal program at the Cleveland Clinic Wellness Institute.

Es has written more than 150 scientific articles, and in 1995 he published the results of his long-term research on arresting and reversing coronary artery disease through nutrition in his book *Prevent and Reverse Heart Disease*. He and his wife, Ann Crile Esselstyn, have been following a plant-based diet for more than twenty-six years.

Es began his long-term study because, after performing surgeries on many women with breast cancer, "I wanted to decrease the number of patients rather than simply wait for the next one to arrive."

To that end, Es performed two decades of global research, finding that, wherever people ate a plant-based diet, cancer and cardiovascular disease were rare. "To do the study, we recruited twenty-four patients from the clinic's cardiovascular department, people who had basically been told to go home and prepare for death, and put them on a plant-based diet. Every one of them who followed the diet lived without any more incidents of heart disease."

Es has been preaching the advantages of a plant-based diet ever since, to a slowly growing audience. "It takes time for people to catch on," he says. "But it will happen. The trigger will be larger studies that will be so compelling that specialists will *have* to offer the option of a lifestyle change to patients.

"Sadly, today most doctors treat only the symptoms, not the cause, giving their patients pills, procedures, and operations that are expensive and dangerous. Some of them say, 'Well, patients won't change their diet.' But if you sit with patients for five hours, as we do, and explain exactly what diet does, why, and how, we find that patients *do* change successfully. This kind of care restores the covenant of trust that must exist between the caregiver and the patient, who realizes you are telling him or her absolutely everything you know about the disease so it can be halted, and even reversed. And the patient then feels empowered to do so.

"Cardiovascular disease is a toothless paper tiger that need never exist. And if it does exist, it need never progress. It is a food-borne illness. Change your food, and you change your life."

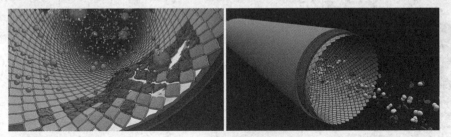

Figure 3a   Figure 3b

Dr. Caldwell Esselstyn's studies have corroborated the concept that the typical Western diet of processed oils, dairy, and meat destroys our endothelial cells (the lining of our blood vessels) and leaves a plaque buildup that inhibits blood flow. Figure 3a shows a blood vessel with plaque buildup; Figure 3b shows the blood vessel of a plant-based eater.

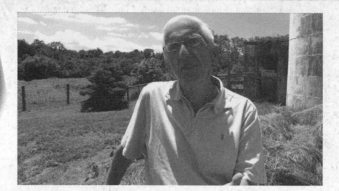

T. Colin Campbell, PhD

T. COLIN CAMPBELL grew up on a dairy farm and was educated at Penn State and Cornell, where, after working on a postdoctoral degree at MIT and teaching at Virginia Tech, he returned for a tenured full professorship in 1975. He has also consulted as a senior science adviser to the American Institute for Cancer Research and currently sits on the advisory board of the Physicians Committee for Responsible Medicine. Since 1978, he has been a member of several National Academy of Sciences expert panels on food and health, and he holds an honorary professorship at the Chinese Academy of Preventive Medicine in Beijing as well as Shanghai Jiao Tong University. Colin is the Jacob Gould Schurman Professor Emeritus of Nutritional Biochemistry at Cornell University and project director of the China-Oxford-Cornell Diet and Health Project.

Colin is best known for the best-selling book *The China Study,* which he coauthored with his son, Thomas M. Campbell, MD. The book represents the culmination of Colin's work as well as his two-decade research partnership with Cornell, Oxford University, and the Chinese Academy of Preventative Medicine. It ties the consumption of animal-protein-based foods to the development of cancer and heart disease, noting that casein, a protein found in milk from mammals, is "the most relevant carcinogen ever identified."

"The study was organized to investigate why cancer mortality rates, published in 1981 by Chinese medical academies, were so varied in different parts of the country—and to assess what role diet and lifestyle factors might play in these unusual rates of disease.

"It was a huge undertaking—we collected data from 130 villages involving 6,500 adults and their families. What we found, based on evaluation of the complex relationship between multiple diet and lifestyle factors, was that the consumption of whole, plant-based foods offered the best strategy for creating health and preventing serious diseases.

"The reception to these findings was generally positive, although there were some negative reports. I was often at the center of this debate—which resulted in some serious consequences.

"The more this went on, the more I learned how deeply connected science is to industry. Accusations about my personal life and my ethics continued, even one that said I had taken my NIH money for personal use, which was a terrible lie. Another example occurred at Cornell, where I was teaching a well-received course on plant-based nutrition. Then, when our book was published and I took a year off to lecture, the course was arbitrarily taken off the books by the department director, who was a consultant for the dairy industry.

"Despite these difficulties, I'm optimistic. The more this information is out there, and the more people experience its benefits, the more the public will change its ways. The horse is out of the barn, as we used to say on the farm."

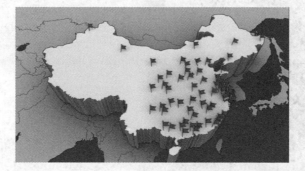

Figure 4: In 1980, Dr. Junshi Chen, currently Senior Research Professor with the Chinese Center for Disease Control and Prevention, teamed with Colin Campbell to create what the *New York Times* called "the most comprehensive large study ever undertaken of the relationship between diet and the risk of developing disease." More than 350 workers were trained to study 6,500 people in 65 counties scattered across China (see above). The results, published in the book *The China Study,* found that the scientific evidence was clear: Whole, plant-based foods were beneficial to human health, while animal-based foods were not.

Cancer

Next to heart disease, cancer is the leading cause of death among Americans; nearly one in three people will develop the disease in their lifetime. Cancer can progress in the body undetected for years, and many cancers are ultimately fatal in spite of expensive interventions like surgery and drugs.

How does your body develop cancer? A normal cell divides and redivides over the course of its life until its telomeres (a telomere is a DNA sequence that lies at the end of a chromosome) are shortened to the point where reproduction is no longer possible. Shortly thereafter, the cell dies. However, some cells may mutate during this process, which can set the stage for cancer development. These mutated cells often reproduce much more rapidly than normal cells, forming tumors and even metastasizing to other parts of the body.

While an individual may be genetically susceptible to cancer, diet and lifestyle choices play a much larger role in whether or not a person will develop it. Some components of food, like animal protein, are powerful cancer promoters. Dairy foods in particular increase the risk of cancer because consuming them causes increased production of a hormone called "insulin-like growth factor" (IGF-1). Higher levels of IGF-1 cause higher levels of estrogen in women and testosterone in men, and abnormal levels of these hormones are responsible for most breast and prostate cancers.

On the other hand, plant-based foods are filled with nutrients like phytochemicals and antioxidants that can fight cancer. Eating these foods can help your body repair mutated cells, or cause apoptosis (death of the cells), reducing your risk of developing cancer.

Diabetes

The number of reported cases of type 2 diabetes, which accounts for 90 to 95 percent of diabetes cases, is growing at an alarming rate. According to the Centers for Disease Control and Prevention, there are currently 25.8 million diabetics in the United States; 79 million more people suffer from pre-diabetes. Much of this growth rate is due to the increased incidence of diabetes in children. In fact, young people account for 45 percent of new type 2 diabetics.

As a result, the disease that used to be called "*adult onset* diabetes" is now simply labeled "type 2 diabetes." Today, some 186,300 Americans under the age of twenty have this form of the disease, and 2 million adolescents between the ages of twelve and nineteen have pre-diabetes. The cost to treat the disease increases by an additional $8 billion every year.

The common view of diabetes is that it develops because of eating too much sugar, but this is not the case. As Dr. Neal Barnard explains, with type 2 diabetes, the body still produces insulin—the hormone that escorts glucose into the cells so it can be used for energy—but the cells develop insulin resistance. Because the cells resist the action of insulin, glucose cannot enter the cells and builds up in the bloodstream. This in turn can cause serious complications.

Why does this resistance happen? Because the cells have become clogged with lipids, or fats. The benefit of switching to a low-fat, plant-based diet is that it causes the cells to release this excess fat, which in turn allows insulin to function normally again. Thus, the solution to insulin resistance is to eat a low-fat, plant-based diet. Countries where people consume a diet based on healthy, high-carbohydrate foods have the lowest diabetes rates in the world.

Dr. Barnard's own research on dietary intervention for diabetes validates the effectiveness of this diet: Patients who were put on a low-fat, plant-based diet experienced greater improvement in their diabetic condition than those placed on a traditional diabetes-management diet, which continues to allow meat and dairy products.

Alzheimer's Disease

Although it doesn't receive as much attention as higher-profile diseases like cancer, Alzheimer's disease can be the most hellish. Alzheimer's patients exhibit few, if any, symptoms at first, but the disease slowly turns into full-fledged dementia. Not only do Alzheimer's patients suffer from the disease, the disease can persist for a very long time, which can be terribly difficult for family members who become caregivers. This is why preventative measures are so crucial.

Alzheimer's is another manifestation of poor cardiovascular health. Studies show that even moderately high cholesterol levels in people in their forties can significantly increase the risk of developing Alzheimer's later in life: One study showed that for those with cholesterol levels between 200 and 239, the risk of developing dementia increased by 52 percent, and for those with levels of 240 or higher, the risk was increased by 66 percent.

Research has yet to produce a cure for Alzheimer's, but studies have consistently demonstrated the virtues of a preventative plant-based diet. During the July 2000 World Alzheimer's Congress, for instance, researchers released the results of a study undertaken between 1993 and 1999 that examined 5,395 individuals aged fifty-five years and older. "On average," the report concluded,

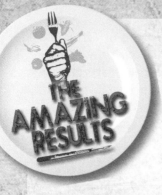

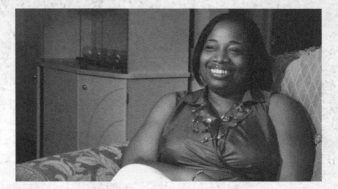

San'Dera

WHEN SAN'DERA PRUDE*, a hospital administrator in Cleveland, Ohio, was in her late thirties, she came down with nagging symptoms—chills, sweating, dizziness, the shakes—and endured them for several months before she decided to consult a doctor. The physician informed her that she had hypertension (i.e., high blood pressure) and diabetes, then handed her a prescription and told her to "watch what you eat."

San'Dera left the doctor's office with no idea what she was supposed to be "watching"—and in any case, it probably didn't matter because she was in deep denial about her condition. She relied on her pills to offset any symptoms and continued eating whatever she wanted whenever she wanted it, causing her to gain a great deal of weight, which made her uncomfortable and depressed.

Struggling to lose her extra pounds, San'Dera tried several crash diets but always ended up going back to her usual fare of scrambled eggs with cheese, sausage, bacon, French toast, and fast-food burgers and quick, fat-laden meals from the cafeteria at work.

San'Dera was desperate to break the cycle of overeating caused by the stress of her diagnosis and her depression. One day she prayed, "You've got to do something, you've got to do something. Lord, help me." And the next day San'Dera was approached to be part of a documentary about the power of dietary intervention (i.e., *Forks Over Knives*) and was referred to Dr. Caldwell B. Esselstyn, Jr.

---

*Before her marriage, she appeared in the film *Forks Over Knives* as San'Dera Nation.

Dr. Esselstyn recommended that San'Dera give up meat, dairy, and processed foods and start on a whole-food, plant-based diet with no refined sugar or added oils. This was a tall order, given her dietary habits, but San'Dera agreed to do it—and to meet often with Dr. Esselstyn. Within a few weeks, she felt better than she had in years, and her blood-sugar levels had returned to normal. By the time the filming was over, San'Dera's symptoms had disappeared, and she had discontinued all of her medications. Even better, her new husband has joined her on the diet and not only has lost weight but was able to discontinue his own diabetes medications.

"people who remained free from any form of dementia had consumed higher amounts of beta-carotene, vitamin C, vitamin E, and vegetables than the people in the study who developed Alzheimer's."

Erectile Dysfunction

Unfortunately, more and more men are suffering from erectile dysfunction at younger and younger ages. Drug companies have built a billion-dollar business around this condition. Just one Viagra pill can cost as much as $15. Using Viagra twice a week can cost as much as $1500 per year, and as yet there are no generic versions of the best-selling drugs available. In spite of their expense, these drugs don't always work; half of the men who take them report that they are ineffective. And the side effects include stomach discomfort, bladder pain, bloody urine, dizziness, diarrhea, and pain during urination.

Erectile dysfunction is often the first symptom of cardiovascular disease. Dr. Terry Mason calls it "the canary in the coal mine" letting you know that you have vascular disease. And, as Dr. Mason says, "If you have vascular disease anywhere, you have it everywhere."

A plant-based diet is not only much less expensive than Viagra and similar drugs, but it usually results in a permanent solution to erectile dysfunction without any negative side effects. There are remarkable benefits to be enjoyed from eating well!

Many other conditions are affected by diet. A final one to consider here is excess weight, which ranks among America's most visible—and most dangerous—epidemics. An expanding waistline is a significant factor in four leading causes of death: heart disease, stroke, diabetes, and cancer. The same unhealthy diets that cause obesity promote plaque formation in blood passageways, the key factor for a heart attack or stroke. Moreover, the National Cancer Institute concluded that many forms of cancer, particularly colon, breast, endometrial, kidney, and esophageal, are directly linked to obesity.

Modern medicine has made little progress in treating common degenerative conditions. Every year, millions of people die from diseases that are completely avoidable; over one million Americans die every year just from heart disease and cancer. But the reality is that most of these ailments are preventable and even treatable through simple lifestyle choices.

The fact that so many diseases are dependent on diet is the reason why, for health and healing, it is far better to rely on food (i.e., your fork) than surgery (i.e., the surgeon's knife). Simply put: Forks over knives.

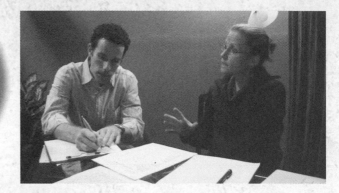

Alona Pulde, MD, and Matthew Lederman, MD

ALONA PULDE, a California native, always wanted to be a doctor: "Maybe that had something to do with the doctor's kit my parents gave me for my fourth birthday." She completed her premedical training at UCLA in 1996; later, her interest in alternative treatments led her to pursue a master's degree in traditional Chinese medicine. She then completed a doctor of medicine in family practice at Albany Medical College in 2004.

When Alona was thirty years old, her father passed away. "With all my training and all my knowledge, I could not understand for the life of me how a healthy man like my dad could suddenly die of a heart attack at age fifty-five," she says. Reading the works of Colin Campbell and Drs. John McDougall and Caldwell Esselstyn on the relationship between diet and health, she came to realize and promote the importance of a low-fat, whole-foods, plant-based diet as an integral part of the medical practice that she had created with her husband, Matt. Today, the couple is working with Whole Foods Market to help develop and oversee the implementation of the company's health and wellness programs.

Matt, who is a physician certified in internal medicine specializing in nutrition and lifestyle medicine, grew up outside Philadelphia and holds a bachelor of science from the University of Michigan and a doctor of medicine from Temple University School of Medicine. Like his wife, Matt "never really considered any other profession" than medicine. "I had always thought I was going to be a cardiologist, just like my father. But I grew disillusioned. The medicine I was practicing had very little to do with actually healing people, which was my original motivation to become a doctor."

Say Alona and Matt, "If you don't switch to a plant-based diet, you will significantly increase your risk of disease. Simply put, you will be more ill and you will die younger.

"People who don't switch run the risk of becoming very overweight and severely de-conditioned. It's only a matter of time before they succumb to one or more chronic diseases. Is the standard American diet really worth a slow, painful death from diabetes? Decreased motor function from debilitating arthritis? Exacerbating cancers of the colon, breast, prostate, and more? A heart attack? Or ending up on countless medications, all with their endless lists of side effects? Why risk ministrokes, small strokes big enough to cause changes in your cognitive functions, or worse, larger strokes able to rob you of your ability to function and interact with your loved ones forever?

"Following the American diet is your one-way ticket to a slow, painful death that often begins in what should very well be the prime of your life. Or, you can switch to a plant-based diet and stop this runaway train in its tracks."

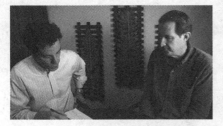

Lee Fulkerson is the writer and director of *Forks Over Knives*. A self-admitted "non-healthy eater," he consulted with Drs. Matt Lederman and Alona Pulde, who immediately put him on a plant-based diet. Below are the results: After thirteen weeks, Lee lost 20 pounds, his blood pressure dropped significantly, his total cholesterol went from 241 to 154, and his LDL (or bad cholesterol) dropped from 157 to 80.

Lee Fulkerson's test results before and after 13 weeks on a whole-foods, plant-based diet

	BEFORE	AFTER
Weight	231 pounds	211 pounds
Blood pressure	142/82	112/70
Resting pulse	92	60
Total cholesterol	241	154
LDL	157	80
CRP*	6	2.8

*This measures inflammation in the heart and blood vessels.

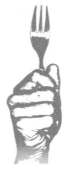

GOOD FOR ANIMALS

Clearly, the impact of a plant-based diet on human health is powerful. But our diet has other effects beyond personal health, raising issues about humankind's relationship with animals, particularly how we treat those animals we have domesticated for our own purposes and those we capture in the wild for food.

ANIMAL FARMS

Life on the farm once conjured up images of sunburned, cheerful farmers tending to vast tracts of rolling pasture, with chickens roaming freely around the barn, pecking at fresh grain and laying eggs at their whim, while the family cow wanders near the henhouse, the silver bell tied around her neck clanging lazily.

Farming has changed. For the sake of maximizing profits and streamlining production, most of today's meat originates in factory-style farms, enormous industrial warehouses crammed with thousands of turkeys, chickens, cows, pigs, or other animals. These suppliers strive to maximize efficiency by raising large numbers of these animals in a short amount of time.

It once took about two years for a calf to grow to the size required for slaughter. In the eyes of a corporation, this growth period represents a substantial overhead cost, because the animals must be fed constantly and treated for disease. In order to reduce this growth period, most factory farms employ artificial growth promotants, such as rBGH (recombinant bovine growth hormone), which allow animals to develop muscle far faster than normal. Although the European Union has banned the use of growth-promoting hormones, approximately two thirds of all beef cattle in the United States are treated with them. In fact, the United States is the only developed nation that permits the use of rBGH for increasing milk production in dairy cows.

Sadly, animals in factory farms are pushed to their biological limits and subjected to tremendous amounts of stress. Like other factory-farmed animals, milk cows endure grueling demands and are susceptible to disease and fatigue. By giving the cows high-energy food and injecting them with growth hormones, farmers can get more milk from their cows. The average cow today produces nearly one hundred pounds of milk per day, ten times what she would produce naturally. Although cows can live twenty or more years, many factory-bred cows can barely walk by their fourth birthday.

Hens exploited for egg production are commonly packed in cages so tightly that they cannot move or even flap their wings. The harsh wire cages are lined up in rows and stacked in tiers in huge factory warehouses. When just chicks, they are subjected to a process known as debeaking, a procedure that involves severing bone, cartilage, and tissue to remove part of the beak—a necessary precaution in many factory farms where severely overcrowded cages provoke pecking and fighting.

Calves raised for veal are typically separated from their mothers immediately after birth and confined thereafter in crates measuring just two feet wide, their movements restrained with neck chains. Males are castrated without painkillers.

Because the cost of every square inch of space is carefully calculated for optimal profits, pigs, too, are packed together tightly, constantly breathing the noxious gases from their own excrement.

At the slaughterhouse, fully conscious chickens are hung by their feet from shackles—because poultry is excluded from the rules of the Humane Methods of Livestock Slaughter Act, stunning them prior to slaughter is not required. If the automated cutter fails to cut their throats, they are killed by other means, or submerged alive in the scalding tank that is used to loosen their feathers so they can be removed later.

All in all, in 2008 the number of animals killed to satisfy American palates was 8.56 billion, or 29 animals per average American meat eater. The total number of animals killed on land and sea was approximately 80 billion, or 270 per American meat and fish eater—making the average number of

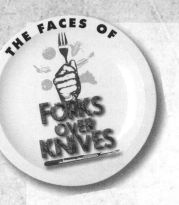

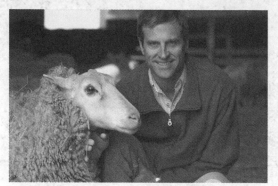

Gene Baur

GENE BAUR, A native Angeleno, graduated from California State University, Northridge, in 1985 and later received a master's degree in agricultural economics from Cornell. The cofounder and president of Farm Sanctuary, America's leading farm-animal protection organization, he is the author of the best-selling book *Farm Sanctuary: Changing Hearts and Minds About Animals and Food*. Gene has photographed and video recorded hundreds of farms, stockyards, and slaughterhouses to expose countless examples of factory-farming cruelty; his work has been featured throughout the major news media.

Gene has also helped initiate legislation to prevent farm-animal abuse by testifying in court and before local, state, and federal legislative bodies; he played an important role in passing the first U.S. laws to prohibit cruel farming methods, including the Florida ban on gestation crates, the Arizona ban on veal calf and gestation crates, and the California ban on foie gras.

From a young age, Gene knew he wanted to help others. "My parents are very conservative Catholics and I grew up with a strong dose of Catholic morality," he recalls. "Not all of it stuck, but some of the basics, like 'Thou shalt not kill' remained important—and these values, enhanced by the folk music I discovered during high school, stuck with me."

So during high school, Gene volunteered with terminally ill kids at children's hospitals; in college, he worked with troubled adolescents and, later, with environmental and public interest groups. Eventually Gene became involved in the nascent movement promoting the ethical treatment of animals and, with his wife at the time, founded Farm Sanctuary. "By the mid-1980s, this was the issue that meant the most to me—and one that was not getting a lot of attention.

"Over the years I have seen terrible things—people being extraordinarily cruel to animals, becoming monsters. I remember once watching some guys at a stockyard using electric prods to move the cows through the pens, and one man was shocking a cow's genitals—inflicting pain just for the fun of it.

"That's one of the scariest things we see—people in the industry engaging in purely sadistic behavior. The people who work at these places don't look at the animals' faces: These animals are nothing but pieces of meat to them. People in slaughterhouses become accustomed to killing, to thinking of violence as normal.

"But it's not all bad news. When we first got our farm in Watkins Glen, New York, a fur farmer lived across the street. We were unhappy about it but were always friendly and invited him to our events. A couple of years later, he came over and told us, 'I don't want to kill animals this way anymore,' and quit the fur business.

"That's what makes the work worthwhile. Visitors come to the farm and leave changed people. They realize that we are what we eat. When we eat meat, we eat misery. These animals know nothing but abject cruelty their whole lives. They are killed in violent ways, and meat eaters ingest that. It's impossible for me to believe that food that is the product of violence and misery can be good for us."

animals consumed in one American lifetime 21,000. While the total number of animals killed to feed Americans has decreased slightly over recent years, the number *slaughtered* in the United States has actually increased because of a rise in U.S. meat exports. (The United States, which has 5 percent of the world's population, accounts for about 20 percent of the animals killed worldwide for food.)

THE PROBLEM WITH FISH

From studies of their sensory systems, including brain structure and functionality, scientists have long understood that fish feel pain and distress. That means that a fish's pain receptors respond much the same way to barbed hooks as those of the anglers who accidentally hook themselves. Wild fish caught in gill nets may be trapped for days; sudden decompression can kill those quickly raised from deep water, and still others don't survive being netted in the first place. Those who make it to the ship's deck alive are left to suffocate or are cut open. Purse-seine nets are used to catch large fish such as tuna, cod, and haddock, who are fully conscious when their gills are slit and their bodies disemboweled. Meanwhile, bottom trawling is one of the most environmentally damaging fishing methods, destroying endangered coral as trawlers indiscriminately scrape the ocean floor much like loggers clear-cutting a forest.

The story is worse for farmed fish: Much like chickens in battery cages, they face high stocking densities that lead to frequent injury and mortality, and they are starved for a week before slaughter in order to clear their intestines. As with land animals used for food, there are no federal welfare regulations for raising or catching fish.

WHAT YOU CAN DO

Two facts are indisputable: The number of farm animals used worldwide for food is growing dramatically, and the treatment of these animals has become increasingly inhumane.

Plant foods, such as grains, legumes, nuts, seeds, fruits and vegetables, are more efficient to produce than animal foods; as a result, the people of the rest of the world consume fewer animal products, per capita, than those of the more affluent countries. That is changing, however, with rising per-capita income and a world population forecasted to grow from 6.5 billion to 9 billion by 2050. As their incomes rise, people are eating more animal products.

The United Nations' Food and Agriculture Organization (FAO) predicts that meat consumption will more than double by 2050, and milk consumption will grow by 80 percent during that period.

The United States has no federal laws to protect farm animals. The Animal Welfare Act of 1970, which set standards for the confinement of animals, exempts animals used for food. And the Humane Slaughter Act doesn't apply to rabbits, fish, or birds, even though chickens represent the vast majority of land animals killed for food in the United States. Most "humane" state laws exempt "standard agricultural practices," which means cruelty is defined not by the degree of suffering inflicted on animals, but by whether this treatment is considered a normal part of farming.

As a result, all the cruel practices mentioned in this chapter are legal.

Animal activists' recent exposure of the extent and magnitude of farm animals' suffering has led to a coordinated response by the animal agriculture lobby at the state level. Their position is well summarized in a *New York Times* article titled "States Look to Ban Efforts to Reveal Farm Abuse" (April 14, 2011). That's not a misprint. Legislators in Florida, Minnesota, and Iowa are working not to ban farm abuse but to ban *revealing* farm abuse.

The best way to reduce the suffering of farm animals is also the best way to improve your own health: Eat a plant-based diet. It's that simple!

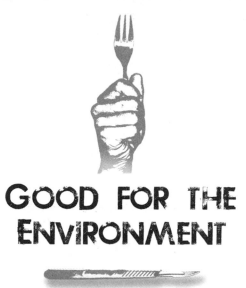

GOOD FOR THE ENVIRONMENT

The conditions under which farm animals are being bred and slaughtered are becoming known to the public—very slowly, and with increasing resistance from the farms themselves. But there are other negative consequences of an animal-based diet, ones that are having larger, planet-wide effects—effects that may well place not just farm animals but the entire planet in jeopardy.

THE TOLLS OF FACTORY FARMING

Global Warming

The United Nations has determined that raising livestock for food purposes generates more climate-heating gases than do all carbon-dioxide-emitting vehicles combined—in other words, cows are worse than cars. Some startling figures: The livestock sector accounts for nearly 10 percent of human-induced carbon dioxide emissions, 37 percent of methane emissions (methane is about 23 times more powerful than CO_2 as a greenhouse gas). It also produces 65 percent of nitrous oxide emissions (nitrous oxide is 296 times more powerful than CO_2) and 64 percent of human-induced ammonia emissions, a significant contributor to acid rain.

While CO_2 is responsible for roughly half of human-related greenhouse gas emissions since the Industrial Revolution, methane and nitrous oxide (both of which are released via livestock's natural digestive processes) are responsible for one third.

Collectively, farm animals themselves are responsible for a fifth of all human-induced greenhouse gases—and this number doesn't include the carbon emissions that result from the massive infrastructure required to transport livestock. A report in *New Scientist* estimated that driving a hybrid car could save about one ton of CO_2 emissions per year but adopting a plant-based diet would save nearly one and a half tons over a comparable period.

According to a recent German study, a meat-centric diet is responsible for the emission of more than seven times as much greenhouse gas as a plant-based diet.

Deforestation

In 2011, livestock operations account for 30 percent of the earth's entire land surface use—much of which has been deforested to create pastureland. For example, nearly 70 percent of deforested land in the Amazon is exploited for grazing, resulting in the destruction of fragile ecosystems and exacerbating excess carbon dioxide in the atmosphere, because unlike standing trees, which capture and store CO_2, felled trees release the gas.

A land area equivalent to seven football fields is destroyed in the Amazon basin every minute. For each hamburger produced from animals raised on rainforest land, approximately 55 square feet of forest have been destroyed.

Waste

Many of these problems are intensified by the inherent inefficiencies of the livestock industry. The process of rearing animals for slaughter is far less efficient than directly harvesting the same crops for human consumption. Studies have shown that a person living exclusively on animal products requires ten times more land than a person growing his or her own plant-based foods.

According to a 1997 report by the Senate Agriculture Committee, animals raised for slaughter produce 130 times as much waste as the entire human population. Our waste is chemically treated in sanitation plants, but animal waste is not: Typically, it is sprayed onto land, then much of it runs off to pollute groundwater or streams.

Water Pollution

A comparable number of issues relate to water usage. The U.S. Environmental Protection Agency estimates that one pound of processed beef requires 2,500 gallons of water. Contrast that with the 250 gallons needed per pound of soy, or the 25 gallons per pound of wheat.

And then there are issues with the water itself. Much of the land harvested exclusively for animal feed is saturated with pesticides and fertilizers used to grow crops as rapidly as possible. These chemicals don't disappear—they seep into groundwater and spill into rivers and oceans. Once in the water they create plumes of toxic chemicals which deplete oxygen in the water, killing fish and other animals.

On top of that, the livestock waste further contaminates the water supply with hormones and antibiotics excreted by the animals.

Then there's the issue of how just how much water it takes to raise animals for food. Worldwide, water use is two to five times greater for crops grown to feed animals than for basic crops. The world's freshwater supply is not evenly distributed, and with increasing demand for water, researchers project that 64 percent of the world's population will live in water-stressed basins by 2025. In the United States, raising animals for food consumes more than half of all the water used, and 80 percent of U.S. freshwater resources are used for agriculture.

All told, the meat industry causes more water pollution in the United States than all other industries combined. According to an article written by Barry Popkin, a professor of nutrition at the University of North Carolina, and published in the *Archives of Internal Medicine*, "In the United States, livestock production accounts for 55 percent of the erosion process, 37 percent of pesticides applied, 50 percent of antibiotics consumed, and a third of total discharge of nitrogen and phosphorus to surface water."

Fisheries Depletion

It's not just the water, but the life within the water that's harmed: Advanced fishing technologies and bottom trawling have led to a massive increase in global fishing, leaving 76 percent of fish stocks either fully exploited, overexploited, or depleted. Given the decimation of desirable wild fish, industry has turned to farmed ones, but these need to be fed: Fishermen are fishing further down the marine food web, catching up to twenty wild fish as feedstock for every single carnivorous fish they raise. As of 2010, the top six types of fish now eaten in the United States are farmed.

Endangered Species

It isn't just fish that are disappearing: Worldwide, we are now losing animal species at a rate that will put us in a state of mass extinction—an event that has occurred five times in the last 540 million years. Top causes include natural habitat destruction, overfishing, hunting, pollution, and desertification. The systematic elimination of whales, wolves, sharks, tigers, mountain lions, and other predators also causes irreversible changes throughout the entire food chain.

We could soon be seeing the sixth mass extinction in the earth's history, and it will be the first one of human origin. Researchers attribute this crisis to "multiple, atypical high-intensity ecological stressors, including rapid, unusual climate change." Extinction of sea life is on the fastest time line: Scientists project that the populations of all commercial fish and seafood species may collapse by 2048.

Soil Erosion

Farms are the leading cause of soil erosion by far, and that erosion—topsoil mixed with agrochemicals and animal waste—leads directly to sedimentation and pollution of watersheds, reservoirs, lakes, and oceans. Approximately 40 percent of the world's agricultural land is seriously degraded, according to scientists at the International Food Policy Research Institute. Animal farming accounts for about 55 percent of soil erosion, and the soil is being depleted at ten to forty times the rate it is being formed. Since cattle began dominating the U.S. plains 140 years ago, more than half of the topsoil in the western United States has been lost.

WHAT YOU CAN DO

According to a 2006 University of Chicago study, the average American diet derives 47 percent of its calories from animal products. This amounts to a carbon "footprint" (i.e., impact) of 2.52 tons of CO_2 emissions per person per year. Those people who are especially partial to red meat—who get, say, 50 percent of their caloric intake from steaks and such—have an average carbon footprint of 3.57 tons.

If the average American meat eater were to reduce his or her intake of animal produce to 25 percent of total calories, it would reduce his or her footprint by approximately one ton. Adopting a purely plant-based diet would mean a two-ton reduction in carbon emissions. In fact, if every American simply reduced chicken consumption by one meal per week, the CO_2 savings would be equivalent to removing 500,000 cars from the road.

Consider this: If the entire U.S. population were to adopt a plant-based diet for just one day, the nation would conserve the following resources[*]:

- 100 billion gallons of drinking water, enough for every person in every home in New England for nearly four months
- 1.5 billion pounds of crops, enough to feed the population of New Mexico for over a year
- 70 million gallons of gasoline, enough to fuel every car in Canada and Mexico
- 33 tons of antibiotics.

Meanwhile, the following environmental damage would be prevented:

- 1.2 million tons of CO_2 greenhouse emissions
- 3 million tons of soil erosion
- 4.5 million tons of animal waste
- 7 tons of ammonia emissions.

Worldwide, farm animals consume 756 million tons of grain. According to Princeton bioethicist Peter Singer, an equivalent amount would be enough to provide the 1.4 billion people living in abject poverty with approximately three pounds of grain per day—twice the amount necessary to survive. Moreover, this figure does not include the 225 million tons of soy produced annually, nearly all of which is consumed by farm animals.

"The world is not running out of food," Singer writes in his book, *The Life You Can Save.* "The problem is that we—the relatively affluent—have found a way to consume four or five times as much food as would be possible if we were to eat the crops we grow directly."

Albert Einstein summed it up best: "Nothing will benefit human health and increase chances for survival of life on Earth as much as the evolution to a vegetarian diet."

---

*Compiled from scientific reports by Noam Mohr, a physicist with the New York University Polytechnic Institute.

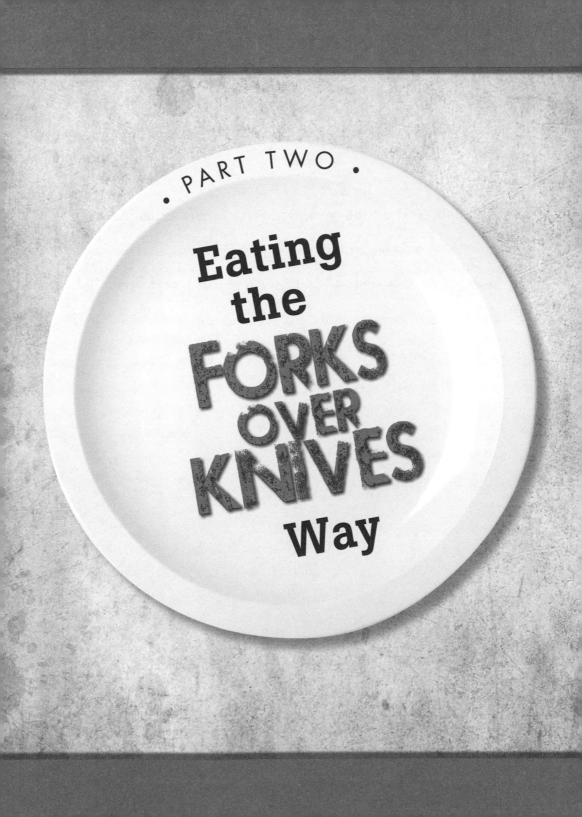

· PART TWO ·

Eating the FORKS OVER KNIVES Way

Now that you know the advantages of a *whole-foods, plant-based* diet, it's time to start cooking whole-foods, plant-based meals. Following are tips you can use to learn more about good nutrition, turn into a smart shopper, stock up your kitchen, and transition to a healthy plant-based diet.

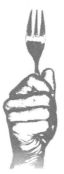

READING NUTRITION LABELS

In an ideal world, everyone would be eating whole foods that arrive without any kind of plastic packaging and, therefore, without that long list of ingredients telling you what's inside—some of it good, most of it bad, and some of it simply mysterious, such as strange compounds that sound less like food and more like something concocted in a chemistry lab.

In the real world, however, even people who have considered themselves to be healthy, whole-plant food eaters for years consume some multi-ingredient foods, which are therefore processed to some degree. Some of these even contain those mystery ingredients.

The ingredient list is the most important piece of text on a product's packaging because it shows, in descending order by weight, everything you are about to put into your body. Be wary of label manipulation. For example, manufacturers often alter their ingredients lists to make it seem as if certain foods are included in lesser quantities than they actually are. This happens most often with sugars. In a practice commonly known as "ingredient splitting," manufacturers use more than one kind of sweetener, such as cane sugar, corn syrup, beet sugar, fructose, and so on, to push what might have been the top-listed ingredient (i.e., heaps of sugar) further down the list so that healthier ingredients can be listed first.

Likewise, expect the unexpected. Foods that you may imagine to be whole and healthy may not be. For example, you may think that you know which foods are high in sodium and which are low, but look again: A seemingly innocent can of vegetable juice may contain up to half of your daily allowance of salt.

Unwanted foods pop up in unexpected places. Dairy appears more often than you would think in products that may not seem to be dairy foods at all: potato chips, breakfast cereals, tomato sauces, and many other nondairy foods. Even some so-called dairy-free cheeses actually contain cow's milk derivatives. That's because dairy products are listed often using terms that you might not recognize: *casein, whey, whey protein, albumen, caseinate, sodium caseinate, lactose, lactic acid, rennet,* and *rennin,* to name a few.

Also, pay attention to serving size. One of the ways that manufacturers fool consumers into buying their products is to make them seem lighter on calories and fat by reducing the serving size listed on the container.

For instance, there's one product in most people's homes whose label indicates that it contains no fat, and yet it is 100 percent fat. This is cooking spray. The reason cooking spray can be all fat and yet call itself "nonfat" is that, according to the Food and Drug Administration, any food that contains less than a half-gram of fat per serving can be called "fat free." A single serving of cooking spray is one incredibly quick spritz—small enough to be less than a half-gram of fat—but most cooks use more than that. Remember: Cooking spray is just fat under a "fat free" label.

Of course, one way to avoid confusion over food labels is to purchase only whole-plant foods. Broccoli, cabbage, bananas, oats, lentils, and other whole-plant foods need no ingredient lists. However, if they had labels, these would look great!

Food Warning Labels

The great Greek doctor Hippocrates said "Let food be thy medicine and medicine be thy food." Now, imagine if food was actually regulated like medicine: What if food producers had to follow the same requirements the pharmaceutical industry must follow when medical studies tie a product to a significant risk of serious or life-threatening effects?

A platter of **tree nuts, legumes, alliums (onions and garlic), vegetables, fruits, and grains** might carry this warning label:

FOOD FACTS

Active Ingredients
Fiber and essential nutrients, including plant protein, vitamins, minerals, phytochemicals (such as carotenoids, flavonoids, terpenes, sterols, indoles, and phenols) and antioxidants that have shown benefit against certain cancers in experimental studies.

Warnings
ALLERGENS: Contains tree nuts, legumes (peanuts and soybeans), and the grains wheat, rye and barley (which contain gluten, a protein composite).

Purpose
For the promotion of good health. These ingredients may reduce the risk of some forms of cancer, heart disease, stroke, obesity, diabetes, high blood pressure, constipation, osteoporosis and other diet-related chronic diseases.

Directions
ALL AGES: Consume three to five servings per day, raw or cooked.

Other Information
May be stored at room temperature or refrigerated for days to weeks.

Inactive Ingredients
Peels, shells, and other biodegradable materials.

A platter of **meat, fish, and dairy,** on the other hand, would carry a more extensive label that might look something like this:

FOOD FACTS

Active Ingredients
Essential nutrients, including protein, vitamins, minerals, and essential fatty acids.

Warnings

ALLERGENS: Contains milk or milk products, eggs, fish, and shellfish.

ASK A DOCTOR BEFORE USE IF YOU HAVE: Cardiovascular disease, cancer, diabetes, Alzheimer's disease, hypertension, obesity, or osteoporosis, or if you are pregnant or nursing.

BIOLOGICAL AGENTS: All primary food-borne pathogens derive from animals, including:

* **BACTERIA:** *Salmonella, Clostridium perfringens, Campylobacter, Staphylococcus aureus, Shigella, E. coli* O157:H7, *Yersinia enterocolitica,* and *Bacillus cereus,* among others
* **PARASITES:** Parasitic protozoa, roundworms, and tapeworms
* **PRIONS:** These proteins in misfolded form may cause Creutzfeldt-Jakob Disease (CJD) or Variant Creutzfeldt-Jakob Disease (vCJD)
* **VIRUSES:** Rotaviruses, astroviruses, and bovine leukemia viruses.

CHEMICAL AND OTHER ETIOLOGICAL AGENTS: May contain arsenicals, pesticides, mercury, chromium, polybrominated diphenyl ethers (PBDE), dioxins, and chemically related compounds. Meat and meat products may contain slaughter waste, antibiotics, artificial growth hormones, veterinary drug residues, trioxypurine, adrenalin, cholesterol, and fecal matter. Fish and shellfish may contain potent marine biotoxins.

BIOACCUMULATION IN ANIMAL TISSUES: Chemical and other etiological agents build up in fat, so low levels in animal feed can produce harmful concentrations in human foods such as meat (including fish), milk, cheese, and eggs. Tuna and other large fish store more mercury than smaller fish because they live longer and ingest smaller fish who themselves store mercury. The primary means of human exposure to dioxins is through the consumption of animal fats, in which dioxins accumulate. Further bioaccumulation occurs when humans consume these animal products. Women can transmit these toxins to fetuses through placental tissue and to infants through breast milk.

OTHER RISK FACTORS: May increase risk of heart disease, cancer, obesity, iron deficiency, asthma, birth defects, ear infections, stomachaches, bloating, diarrhea, gout, hypercholesterolemia, angina, hypertension, prostate disease, multiple sclerosis, kidney stones, cataracts, osteoporosis, diabetes (I and II), rheumatoid arthritis, macular degeneration, hypertension, acne and other skin conditions, migraine, lupus, depression, Alzheimer's disease, muscular dystrophy, Parkinson's disease, cognitive dysfunction, erectile dysfunction, irritable bowel syndrome, body odor, and bad breath.

GLOBAL PUBLIC HEALTH RISKS: Feeding practices and intensive confinement of genetically similar animals fuel zoonotic pathogen adaptation and restrict animals' evolution for resistance to pathogens. Approximately 73 percent of the emerging human pathogens are transmitted to people from animals. The transfer of multi-drug-resistant pathogens from farms and food to humans (e.g., avian influenza H5N1 and swine flu) constitutes a serious biomedical, public health, and biodefense threat. In the United States, farm animals generate three times more excrement than humans, and this waste contaminates water, land, crops, other vegetation, and the air. A United Nations report names animal agriculture as one of the largest sources of global warming emissions. The public risks from consuming animal products (e.g., infectious diseases, widespread pollution, global warming, and shortages of energy, water, and food) may exceed the personal health risks.

continued

Purpose

To prevent starvation. There are virtually no nutrients in animal-based foods that are not better provided by plants. Reliance solely on animal products may create nutritional deficiencies.

Directions

Ask a doctor or health professional before use.

Wash your hands after coming into contact with animal products, and wash cooking, serving, eating, and food preparation surfaces and utensils after they come into contact with animal products. Keep out of reach of children until properly cooked.

Approximately one in six Americans gets sick from food-borne diseases every year. Follow recommended storage temperatures and maximum storage times before and after cooking. Cook meats to an internal temperature of 165°F or greater. Discard beef suspected to contain bovine spongiform encephalopathy (BSE), as the pathogens cannot be killed via cooking—however, this may not be discoverable, as a single hamburger may contain meat from hundreds of animals, and the USDA has banned private-party BSE testing in the United States. Prion proteins, the precursors of prions, have been discovered in pasteurized milk, and this could represent a risk of exposure to transmissible spongiform encephalopathies (TSE), including BSE. Cooking animal tissues can create known carcinogens. Animal flesh should be sufficiently heated to prevent food poisoning from pathogens, but not heated enough to create excessive cancer-causing agents.

Other Information

Store at 37°F for 2–3 days for most meats, 1 day for seafood, 3–5 days for milk, 2–3 weeks for eggs (in shell); keep all tightly covered and protect from excessive moisture. These are general guidelines only.

Inactive Ingredients

Anticoagulants, antimicrobials, antioxidants, binders, coloring agents, curing accelerators, denuding agents, film forming agents, flavoring agents, packaging systems, pH modifiers, poultry scald agents, and tenderizing agents.

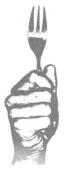

Your Guide to Plant-Based Foods

When people change their diet, they often become focused on what they *can't* eat instead of what they can. Here is a general list of just some of the many wonderful foods that will be part of your diet once you follow the *Forks Over Knives* path.

These suggestions are just that: suggestions. The more you explore the world of plant-based, whole foods, the more you'll enjoy eating things you may never have heard of before—vegetables such as cardoon, Chinese broccoli, lotus root, and tomatillo, and fruits such as carambola, cherimoya, longan, mangosteen, monster, and sapote. Soon you'll be making suggestions to other people, recommending favorite foods that you may not even know about yet.

▶ **FOODS TO EAT FREELY**

Fruits and Vegetables

Fruits—Including apples, apricots, bananas, berries, citrus, dates, figs, grapes, mangoes, melons, peaches, pears, pineapple, plums, and pomegranates

Vegetables—Including asparagus, carrots, celery, cucumbers, onions, peppers, pumpkin, sweet potatoes, tomatoes, and squash (yes, some of these are botanically fruit, but we think of them as vegetables)

Cruciferous vegetables—Including broccoli, Brussels sprouts, cabbage, cauliflower, radishes, Swiss chard, turnips, and watercress

Leafy greens—Including beet greens, chard, collards, kale, lettuce, parsley, and spinach

Sprouts—Including adzuki bean, alfalfa, broccoli, mung bean, soybean, and sunflower

Tubers—Including parsnips, potatoes, and yams

Mushrooms

Including cremini, portobello, shiitake, and other mushrooms

Legumes

Including beans, chickpeas, lentils, and peas

Whole Grains

Including amaranth, barley, corn, kasha, millet, oats, quinoa, rice, and wheat berries

▶ **FOODS TO EAT MORE SPARINGLY**

Avocados
Coconut
Dried fruits
Nuts and seeds
Olives

▶ **LIGHTLY PROCESSED/INSTANT/READY-MADE FOODS THAT ARE OKAY TO EAT**

Pasta sauces—Choose sauces with little to no added oils.

Plant milks—These include soy, rice, oat, hemp, and nut milks, such as almond milk.

Oil-free salad dressings—Dressings should also be low in added sweetners.

Soups made with whole foods—They can be canned or dried. (Dr. Mc-Dougall's line of light-sodium soups is particularly good.)

Whole-grain breads, mixes, and crackers—These include whole-grain bagels, cereals, muffins, pancakes, pastas, pita pockets, pizza crusts, and waffles. Be careful to avoid added oils, sugars, and other unwanted ingredients.

▶ WHICH FOODS ARE CONCENTRATED SOURCES OF VITAMIN C? POTASSIUM? CALCIUM?

Every day, we see messages saying things like, "Calcium is good for your bones" or "Vitamin C helps to prevent colds." These statements and others like them fuel an interest in individual nutrients and can cause people to seek out certain foods because they contain more of a particular vitamin or mineral than other foods.

This is a misdirected strategy because optimal health cannot be achieved by focusing on a few nutrients or eating a few special foods that contain more iron or potassium. In fact, many people experience frustration because they have added or eliminated foods, or increased their consumption of a particular nutrient, without noticing much improvement in their weight or health.

The reason for this frustration is that good health can only be achieved by focusing on adopting a healthful dietary pattern: a low-fat, plant-based diet comprised of whole foods.

So don't worry about eating a particular food in order to get enough of a certain vitamin and instead focus on eating a wide variety of fruits, vegetables, legumes, and whole grains.

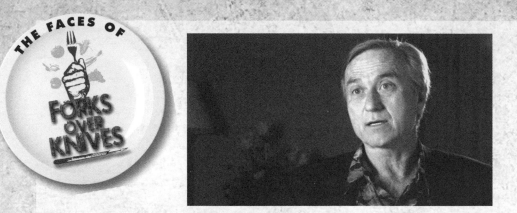

John A. McDougall, MD

DR. JOHN A. MCDOUGALL, who has been studying and writing about the effects of nutrition on disease for more than thirty years, is the founder and medical director of the McDougall Program, a ten-day residential treatment program located in Santa Rosa, California, that features a low-fat, starch-based diet.

A Michigan native, John graduated from Michigan State University's College of Human Medicine and received an MD in 1972 from Queen's Medical Center in Honolulu, where he also performed his internship, and did his residency in internal medicine at the University of Hawaii. He is the author of several national best sellers, including his latest book, *The McDougall Program for a Healthy Heart,* and cofounder and chairman of Dr. McDougall's Right Foods, Inc., a line of plant-based convenience meals made with no added oils and less than 10 percent of their calories derived from fat.

John has dedicated his life to urging the public to eat a high-starch, plant-based diet.

"It started in 1972, when I went to Hawaii to do my medical internship and took a job at a sugar plantation, where I was the primary doctor for five thousand people. On that plantation were workers of Japanese, Filipino, Korean, and other Asian descent. Soon I learned my limitations as I tried, and often failed, to help these people cope with chronic diseases using pills and surgeries.

"I also noticed that my patients spanned four generations, and observed how members in each one ate differently. The older generations consumed mostly rice and vegetables, just as they had in their native lands. Their children's diets were becoming more Westernized. I eventually realized that as soon as people move from a dairy- and meat-free diet to one that includes animal foods, they become ill.

"In 1976, while studying at the University of Hawaii, I began to put into practice the lessons I'd learned. I asked patients to get off oils and switch to a high-starch diet, and the results were immediate.

"Given the excellent results, I was sure that everyone else would see, and do, as I did. That didn't happen. Instead, I was horrified to watch Americans being urged to eat a diet full of meat and dairy. Not surprisingly, they became sicker and sicker. It's been disappointing, but large financial interests are keeping the truth from the public. There just isn't the same kind of money behind promoting starches like corn and potatoes as there is promoting meat and dairy.

"In the 1980s, when my books started coming out, I thought my ideas were going to change America and the world. It didn't happen that way. In fact, it got so bad that my publishers actually told me that they wanted me to change my focus and write about high-protein, low-carb diets, or they'd stop publishing me.

"I laughed at them—and then came Atkins and other enormously successful meat-based, low-carb diets. But now we're in the 2010s, and things have changed. Frankly, I think I'm going to have the last laugh."

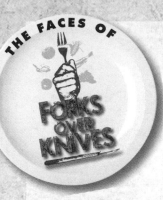

THE FACES OF

FORKS OVER KNIVES

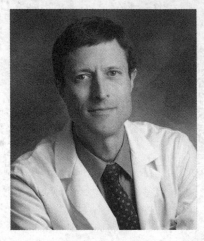

Neal Barnard, MD

DR. NEAL BARNARD is an adjunct associate professor of medicine at the George Washington University in Washington, D.C., and a researcher funded by the National Institutes of Health. He is also the editor-in-chief of the *Nutrition Guide for Clinicians* and the author of more than fifteen books on nutrition and health as well as numerous journal articles.

Neal received his doctor of medicine and completed his residency at George Washington, then practiced at St. Vincent's Hospital in New York City before returning to Washington in 1985 to found the Physicians Committee for Responsible Medicine (PCRM), a nationwide group of physicians and supporters that promotes preventative medicine and addresses controversies in modern health care. In 1991, Neal initiated the Cancer Project, which provides nutritional information for cancer prevention and survival, and later he founded the Washington Center for Clinical Research, a center for nutrition-related studies.

While he was still in college, Neal decided to become a doctor. The year before starting medical school, he worked as an autopsy assistant at a Minneapolis hospital. One day, the pathologist in charge was attending to a man who'd died from a massive heart attack; he removed a wedge of ribs from the man's chest and placed it on the table, pointing out to Neal the atherosclerosis (i.e., fatty buildup inside the arteries) visible in the heart. The doctor told Neal this condition was caused by Americans' bacon-and-eggs lifestyle. At the end of the examination, Neal put the ribs back in the man's chest and went to the hospital cafeteria—to find that lunch that day was spareribs.

"They looked and smelled just like the body I'd just seen," he recalls. "I couldn't eat them. It preyed on my mind, and the connections between what we eat and our health became clearer and clearer to me."

Neal began to realize that "[although Western medicine is] good at diagnosis and treatment, it is abysmal at prevention. I felt it was important for doctors to become advocates and teachers. That's why I set up PCRM."

"Nutrition is critical for health. Many Americans are taking numerous medications three to four times a day, yet they haven't changed the dietary regimen that made them sick in the first place. Most people are not aware that these foods are, if anything, more powerful than the drugs.

"If we cut our skin or break a bone, we take it for granted that the body will heal. But we can also heal from heart disease, weight problems, and diabetes—yet that will never happen if we do not we get away from the foods that are causing the problem and take advantage of foods that heal.

"Currently, conventional treatment for a person with diabetes or hypertension is medications; he or she might or might not be told about a plant-based diet as an 'alternative.' We should turn that around, addressing the diet first— after all, diet is often the cause of the problem—and then, if needed, adding medications. A plant-based diet has the power to reverse heart disease and diabetes and to restore people to health. The sooner it begins, the better off the patient is going to be."

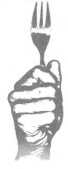

TIPS FOR TRANSITIONING

Changing your diet—whether that means starting on a new path of plant-based eating, simply cutting back on meat and dairy and adding more plant-based foods, or perhaps refining your habits to eliminate processed oils—takes commitment and dedication.

In his book *21-Day Weight Loss Kickstart*, Dr. Neal Barnard suggests an interesting approach for switching to plant-based foods: He recommends that you make a list of the meals you like the most, then go through that list and tweak it. For example, remove the butter from the toast and replace it with sugarless jam, take the butter out of the oatmeal and add blueberries, take the butter off the pancakes, and, while you're at it, add whole wheat flour to the batter.

▶ **FOR BREAKFAST.** There are plenty of plant-based milk substitutes to eat with your whole-grain cereal, but don't be tied to tradition. Smoothies make fantastic breakfasts, and you can make them out of almost anything. Leftovers can also make a wonderful start to the day. Many Asian cultures traditionally eat soup for breakfast. Why not give it a try?

▶ **PREPARING SAVORY DISHES.** Often the delicious smells and tastes that people attribute to animal foods come at least as much from the onion, garlic, mushrooms, and other vegetables that they have been cooked with. Use vegetable broth, water, lemon juice, or other liquids for "sautéing" foods to get the flavor without the fat. Add chopped onion, carrot, and celery to cooking grains. Slow-cooking casseroles and stews can make it easy to achieve deep, complex flavors.

► **MAKING SAUCES AND DRESSINGS.** Mushrooms can be used to make extremely flavorful gravy. Soup can be used as a sauce on top of grains or baked potatoes. Possibilities for salad dressings are endless: Try using pureed whole fruit such as oranges or grapefruit to make them thicker without the oil.

► **MAKING SOUPS.** After cooking soup, blend at least part of it and pour the pureed liquid back into the pot to make a creamy base. The thicker texture will make it taste richer.

► **FOR SNACKS AND DESSERTS.** There are many delicious snack and dessert recipes in this book, but do remember that simple foods can be the perfect choice. Satisfy your sweet cravings or lift your late-afternoon lag with fresh fruit. Keep cut vegetables in the fridge and oil-free hummus and crackers on hand. Bring snacks like these with you in the car, to work, and on errands.

HERE ARE SOME tools that will help you to prepare easy, delicious, healthy, plant-based meals:

▶ **BLENDER.** Handy for making smoothies or combining mostly liquid ingredients. Because of the toughness of kale and some other green vegetables, consider buying a blender with a strong motor, such as a Blendtec or Vitamix.

▶ **CITRUS REAMER.** Very useful if you like using juice from fresh citrus fruits.

▶ **COLANDER.** Perfect for draining steamed vegetables and rinsing berries or beans.

▶ **COOKIE SHEETS.** For baking healthy whole-grain cookies.

▶ **COOLING RACKS.** For cooling baked goods.

▶ **CROCK-POT OR SLOW-COOKER.** A great appliance for making soups, stews, and casseroles. Just add all the ingredients, turn it on, and forget about it!

▶ **CUTTING BOARD.** You will get a lot of use out of this kitchen staple. Choose wood or plastic, whatever your preference. On a plant-based diet there is no need for concern about cross-contamination among raw foods.

▶ **FOOD PROCESSOR.** Absolutely essential for making dips, dressing, spreads, sauces, and other thicker-consistency condiments.

▶ **GLASS BOWLS.** For mixing ingredients for baking, marinades, and so on. Those with lids are convenient for storage.

▶ **GLASS COUNTERTOP CANISTERS WITH LIDS.** For storing everything from flour to dried beans.

- ▶ **IMMERSION BLENDER.** This is a handy tool for making creamy soups or blending hot liquids. You can combine ingredients right in the pot, without the mess or danger of transferring hot soup in batches between the pot and a conventional blender.

- ▶ **KNIVES.** You really only need one good long knife—find one that you really like, and keep it sharp. You'll also want a small knife and a short, serrated knife—these are key for cutting avocados, mangoes, and other whole foods that require some dexterity.

- ▶ **MANDOLINE.** Not essential, but very useful for cutting vegetables. Many mandolines have multiple settings for different thicknesses and cuts.

- ▶ **MEASURING CUPS AND SPOONS.** In various sizes: ¼-cup, ⅓-cup, and ½-cup measuring cups, a 2- or 4- cup glass measuring cup, and a 1-cup glass measuring cup with a spout, for liquids. Also ¼-teaspoon, ½-teaspoon, 1-teaspoon, and 1-tablespoon measuring spoons.

- ▶ **MIXING UTENSILS.** Including wire whisks in different sizes.

- ▶ **PARCHMENT PAPER.** For occasional oil-free brownies and cookies.

- ▶ **PIZZA STONE, WOODEN PIZZA PEEL, AND PIZZA CUTTER.** To make great plant-based, cheese-free pizzas!

- ▶ **POTS AND PANS.** In various sizes for everything from bread, brown rice, and soups to stir fry: 1-, 2-, 4-, and 8-quart saucepans with covers, a 12-inch skillet with a cover, and a 9-inch square cake pan, 9 × 13-inch baking pan, and 9 × 5-inch loaf pan.

- ▶ **RICE COOKER.** Cooks any grain perfectly: brown rice, quinoa, barley, and more. Just throw any of them in with the right amount of water and go for a jog or drive a carpool—when you get home, dinner will be done!

- ▶ **ROLLING PIN.** For making your own whole-wheat pizza dough or healthy cookie dough.

▶ **SCISSORS.** Useful for more things than you can imagine, including opening tofu containers, snipping cilantro, preparing whole peeled tomatoes, and more. Wash them in the dishwasher just like a knife.

▶ **SPATULAS.** At least one straight spatula, one spatula with an angled handle, and one rubber scraper spatula.

▶ **SPICE RACK.** Should include a variety of spices and herbs, including sweet and savory flavors.

▶ **SPOONS.** Including a slotted spoon, a wooden spoon, a sturdy metal spoon, and a soup ladle.

▶ **STEAMING BASKET OR BAMBOO STEAMER.** Steaming is the best way to cook vegetables.

▶ **VEGETABLE PEELER.** Makes short work of peeling everything from potatoes to butternut squash. Some vegetable peelers come with various blade attachments such as julienne, crinkle cut, and slicing.

▶ **WHISK.** For combining baking ingredients and whipping up your own dressings and vinaigrettes.

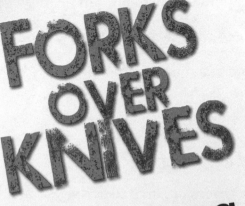

PART THREE

FORKS OVER KNIVES

RECIPES

Now, whether you're already accustomed to a plant-based diet or just starting out, here are 125 recipes to add to your daily repertoire—favorites from a wide range of plant-based cooks and eaters, a number of whom are featured in *Forks Over Knives*.

To learn more about the recipe contributors, see pages 200–202, as well as the "Faces of *Forks Over Knives*" and "The Amazing Results" features throughout this book.

Oatmeal with Fruit

KAREN CAMPBELL | THE CAMPBELL FAMILY

MY HUSBAND, COLIN, likes to have this for breakfast every morning.

SERVES 2

2 cups water

1 cup old-fashioned oats

½ cup raisins

1 cup blueberries

1 cup strawberries

2 kiwis, sliced

1 banana

1 teaspoon maple syrup

1 teaspoon flaxseed meal, optional

1 tablespoon walnuts, optional

1. Bring water to a boil, add oats and raisins, and stir. Cook until thick (2 to 3 minutes).
2. Cut up fruit and mix together. Scoop cooked oatmeal into a bowl. Add maple syrup, walnuts, and flaxseed meal, then fruit.

VARIATION:
▶ Substitute any of the fruits based on your own preferences.

Cinnamon-Raisin Oatmeal

JO STEPANIAK | *BREAKING THE FOOD SEDUCTION* BY NEAL BARNARD, MD

HEARTY, OLD-FASHIONED ROLLED oats in the morning will keep you satisfied until lunchtime. Raisins add a bit of natural sweetness with no added sugar.

SERVES 4

4 cups water
2 cups old-fashioned rolled oats
½ cup raisins
½ teaspoon cinnamon
¼ teaspoon salt
Vanilla soy or rice milk, optional

Combine all ingredients in a heavy saucepan. Bring to a boil, lower heat, and cook, stirring occasionally, for about 10 minutes, or until cooked to your liking. Serve plain or with vanilla soy or rice milk, if desired.

VARIATIONS:

▶ For Cinnamon-Apricot Oatmeal, replace raisins with ½ cup chopped dried apricots. Cook as directed.

▶ For Cinnamon-Apple Oatmeal, reduce water to 3¼ cups and replace raisins with one apple, peeled and coarsely chopped. Cook as directed.

▶ Omit raisins, cook as directed, and top each serving with a dollop (about 1 teaspoon) of fruit-sweetened jam or jelly.

Rip's Big Bowl

RIP ESSELSTYN | *THE ENGINE 2 DIET*

THIS HAS BEEN my mainstay breakfast for more than twenty years. I never get sick of it, and no two bowls are ever quite the same, depending on which fruits are in season and the milk substitute I have on hand. This was also a favorite recipe for most of our Engine 2 Pilot Study participants. As a seven-year-old daughter of one of the participants said, "I look forward to waking up in the morning just so I can have my Rip's Bowl." Let your appetite be your guide as to the size of your bowl.

SERVES 1

¼ cup old-fashioned oats
¼ cup Grape-Nuts or Ezekiel brand equivalent
¼ cup bite-size shredded wheat
¼ Uncle Sam Cereal
1 tablespoon flaxseed meal
2 tablespoons raisins
½ handful of walnuts
1 banana, sliced
1 kiwi, sliced
1 grapefruit
¾ cup plant-based milk (see page 68)

Toss all ingredients except the grapefruit and plant-based milk in a bowl. After cutting the grapefruit in half, use a small, sharp knife to remove the segments. Add the segments to the top of the bowl and squeeze in the juice. Top the bowl with plant-based milk.

TIP ▶ In a pinch, simply add water (the fruits blend with the water and give it a sweet taste).

VARIATION:
▶ Add any fresh or frozen fruit, such as peaches, cherries, mangoes, blueberries, or red grapes.

Blueberry Oat Breakfast Muffins

JULIEANNA HEVER | THE PLANT-BASED DIETITIAN

THESE QUICK AND easy breakfast muffins are a sweet, comforting way to start your day. Picky kid–tested and plant-based Mom approved, these moist, low-fat, fruit-filled delights are great for any occasion!

MAKES 12 MEDIUM MUFFINS

> 1 medium banana, mashed
> One 15-ounce can sweet potato puree
> ¼ cup 100% pure maple syrup
> 1 teaspoon vanilla extract
> 2 cups whole oat flour
> ½ teaspoon baking soda
> ½ teaspoon baking powder
> ½ teaspoon salt
> 1 teaspoon ground cinnamon
> ½ teaspoon ground nutmeg
> ¼ teaspoon ground ginger
> 1 cup fresh or frozen blueberries

1. Preheat the oven to 375°F. In a large bowl, combine the mashed banana, sweet potato puree, maple syrup, and vanilla extract.
2. In a small bowl, combine the oat flour, baking soda, baking powder, salt, cinnamon, nutmeg, and ginger. Transfer the mixture to a large bowl and mix together gently until well combined. Avoid over-mixing to prevent toughness in the final product. Fold in the blueberries.
3. Spoon the batter into silicone muffin cups and bake for 20 minutes or until the muffins are lightly browned. Remove from the oven and let cool for 5 minutes. Store the muffins in an airtight container.

Brian's Awesome Smoothie

BRIAN WENDEL | EXECUTIVE PRODUCER OF *FORKS OVER KNIVES*

I LOVE FRUIT. This is my favorite smoothie, and I never get tired of it. I especially enjoy a smoothie after a rigorous workout.

SERVES 2

> 2 mangoes
> 5 to 6 bananas

Peel and chop the mangoes and bananas. Put all the ingredients in a blender and puree, adding water as needed.

TIP ▶ Try using papaya instead of mango for a refreshing alternative.

Gene's Green Machine Smoothie

GENE BAUR | FOUNDER OF FARM SANCTUARY

SERVES 2

> 2 cups plant-based milk (see page 68)
> 1 banana (optionally frozen)
> ¼ cup frozen blueberries
> 2 large leaves of kale
> ½ cup spinach
> ½ English cucumber (optional)
> ½ tablespoon flax seeds, and/or ½ tablespoon hemp or chia seeds
> 1 date, pitted (optional)
> Ice (optional)

Blend all the ingredients until smooth and no chunks remain. Add more plant-based milk or water to get the consistency you prefer.

Chocolate Smoothie

NO ONE WILL know there are any greens in this smoothie unless you tell them.

MAKES TWO 16-OUNCE SERVINGS

¾ **cup unsweetened almond milk**

½ **cup pomegranate juice**

6 **ounces organic baby spinach, optional**

1 **frozen banana**

Dates (or date paste) to taste

3 **tablespoons raw cocoa powder**

2 **cups frozen blueberries**

Puree all the ingredients in a high-powered blender until smooth.

VARIATION:

▶ When available, I like to use 1 cup blueberries and 1 cup cherries.

Nondairy Milk Alternatives

The soy-milk market has mushroomed over the last three decades, and other milk replacements are becoming mainstream. Those not readily available can be made in your own kitchen. These varieties include grain milks, such as oat, barley, and rice; legume milks, such as peanut and soy; nut milks, such as almond, cashew, coconut, and hazelnut; and seed milks such as hemp, sesame, and sunflower.

Soy milk is a popular choice for topping cold and hot cereals, in coffee and tea, and for cooking, but all plant milks can be delicious, and your individual preferences should dictate. Soy, rice, and almond milk are all good candidates for baking, but those with tree-nut allergies should avoid all nut milks. For a buttermilk replacement, try stirring a tablespoon of white or cider vinegar or lemon juice into a cup of soy milk.

Fresh Almond Milk

CHEF AJ | *UNPROCESSED*

OF COURSE, YOU can buy almond milk at the store, but why not make your own for just pennies a glass? It's really easy and delicious! The only special equipment you'll need is a new paint-straining bag (one that hasn't been used for painting!). You can get one at any hardware store for about 99 cents.

MAKES 3 CUPS

1 cup raw almonds (or your favorite nut or seed)

1. Soak the almonds overnight in filtered water. Be sure to cover completely because they expand as they absorb water.
2. In the morning, drain the almonds completely and rinse well several times. Put the almonds in a blender with 3 cups filtered water. Blend on high speed until the almonds are fully incorporated into the liquid.
3. Place the straining bag, open, in a medium bowl and pour the mixture into the bag. Twist the top of the bag closed and lift it up to let the milk strain into the bowl. Squeeze the bag with your other hand until you can't work any more liquid out of the pulp. You can reserve the pulp for another use such as making cookies or crackers. Any unused milk will keep, refrigerated, for 2 to 3 days.

TIP ▶ If you like your nut milk thicker and richer, more like cream, just add less water. For thinner almond milk, add more water.

VARIATIONS:

▶ For a sweet version, add a few dates (or date paste) and alcohol-free vanilla extract or almond extract.

▶ For an even cheaper, easier version simply add 1–2 teaspoons of raw almond butter to each 1 cup of water and blend until smooth.

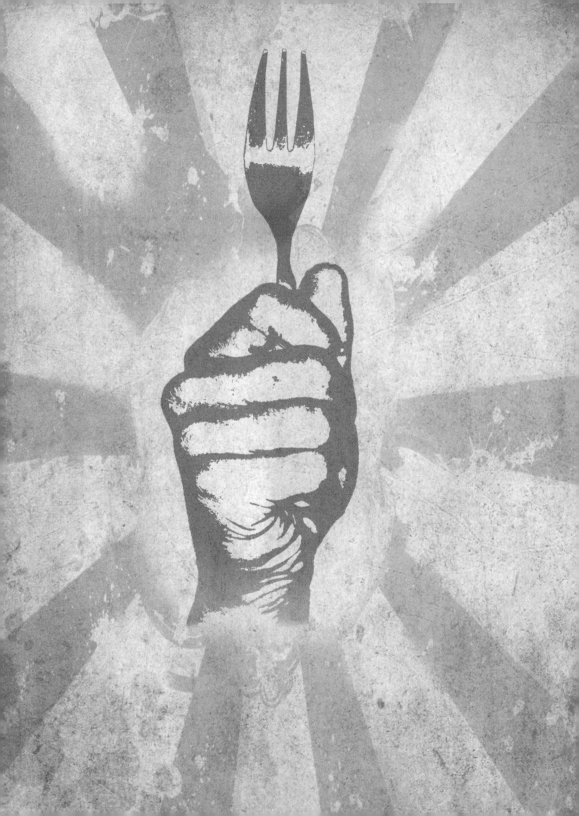

Joey's Lifesaving Sweet Potato Chips

JOEY AUCOIN | FEATURED IN *FORKS OVER KNIVES*

THESE CHIPS ARE my favorite snack, especially at parties when everything else is loaded with oil. They take almost no time to make and everybody loves them. Try serving them with a dressing made from balsamic vinegar, rice syrup, and mustard; with cashew-spinach dip; or with tomato-avocado dip.

Sweet potatoes or potatoes, sliced very thin

Microwave potato slices on high for approximately 7 minutes.

TIP ▶ These will not be as crunchy as fried potato chips, but they're a treat, and definitely stiff enough to put dip on.

Spicy Garbanzo Spread

MARY MCDOUGALL | THE MCDOUGALL PROGRAM

THIS MAKES A delicious sandwich spread or wrap filling, a dip for raw vegetables, or a stuffing for pita bread.

MAKES 1½ CUPS

One 15-ounce can chickpeas, drained and rinsed
2 green onions, chopped
1½ tablespoon grated ginger
1 tablespoon soy sauce
1 teaspoon rice vinegar
½ teaspoon minced fresh garlic
½ teaspoon agave nectar
Sriracha Hot Chili Sauce, optional

Puree all the ingredients except the hot sauce in a food processor until smooth. Add hot sauce if desired and adjust seasonings to taste. Refrigerate at least 1 hour to allow the flavors to blend.

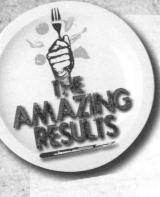

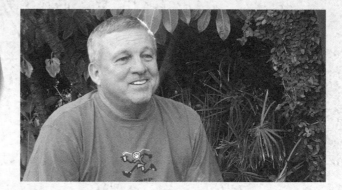

Joey

JOEY AUCOIN, HAPPILY married with three children, always led an active life. A native of Florida, Joey played baseball, fished, swam, rode motorcycles, and never endured any major health issues. He always ate whatever he wanted, seemingly without consequences beyond the supposedly inevitable weight gain seen in middle-aged people.

Then, at age fifty-two, during a trip to New York, Joey began to feel symptoms of high blood sugar—his vision suddenly became clouded, and he began waking up in a cold sweat. He told his wife, "Cammie, when we get home I gotta have my eyes checked. I think I need to get a different prescription because my eyes are just real blurry."

A trip to the doctor settled the question: His blood sugar clocked in at 480, far beyond the level of someone with pre-diabetes or insulin resistance. With almost no warning, Joey had received a diagnosis of full-blown type 2 diabetes.

What followed were years of enslavement to many medications. Joey could never go anywhere without bringing along his shots and pills, some of which needed to be refrigerated. And they were expensive: one hundred dollars a month, out of pocket, plus the frequent cost of overnight mail when he'd forget to take them along while traveling out of town.

More painful than the costs were the side effects. Although the medications controlled his blood sugar, they also caused a laundry list of issues including fatigue, digestive problems, and trouble sleeping.

Then, a friend who was working on the set of *Forks Over Knives* suggested that Joey might want to appear in the film. Soon he was in Los Angeles meeting with Dr. Matt Lederman, who took him off his meat- and dairy-laden diet, prescribing a 100 percent whole-foods, plant-based diet with no added sugar or oils.

Within two days, Joey enjoyed his first good night's sleep in memory. And today, just a few years later, he is healthy, fit, happy, and uses only a tiny fraction of the medication he once needed.

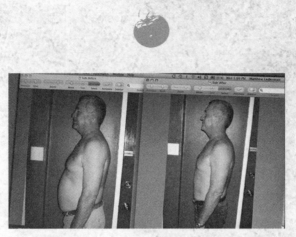

Joey Aucoin lost 28 pounds over the course of 22 weeks.

Pea Guacamole

MARY MCDOUGALL | THE MCDOUGALL PROGRAM

THIS TASTES SO much like the real thing that most people won't be able to guess what it is made from.

MAKES 2 CUPS

2 pounds frozen green peas, thawed
1 teaspoon crushed garlic
¼ cup fresh lime juice
½ teaspoon ground cumin
1 tomato, chopped
4 green onions, chopped
½ cup chopped fresh cilantro
⅛ teaspoon hot pepper sauce
Sea salt

Put the peas, garlic, lime juice, and cumin into the bowl of a food processor and process until smooth. Scrape the mixture into a bowl and stir in the tomato, green onions, cilantro, and hot sauce. Add salt to taste. Cover and refrigerate for at least 30 minutes to allow the flavors to blend.

Eggplant Dip

MATT LEDERMAN AND ALONA PULDE—WITH THANKS TO SHOSHANA PULDE | *KEEP IT SIMPLE, KEEP IT WHOLE*

THE DAYS OF wishing for dairy-free baba ghanoush are past. Enjoy a creamy dip that's great for crackers or cut vegetables or spread in a sandwich.

SERVES 4

5 large eggplants
5 garlic cloves, crushed
Juice of 1 large lemon
1 to 2 tablespoons tahini
5 green onions, chopped
Salt and black pepper

1. Heat the oven or grill to 400°F.
2. Roast the whole eggplants on a baking sheet in the oven or directly on the grill for 40 to 50 minutes until soft; let cool.
3. Scoop out the insides of the eggplants and put them into a bowl; discard the peels. Mash the eggplant, then let stand for about 30 minutes. Discard any accumulated juices.
4. Add the garlic, lemon juice, tahini, and green onions to the eggplant and mix together. Add salt and pepper. Keep covered and refrigerated.

Tofu-Spinach Dip

ALAN GOLDHAMER AND DOUG LISLE | *THE HEALTH PROMOTING COOKBOOK*

KEEP YOUR CREAMY dip without falling back into the Pleasure Trap. Serve as a dip with fresh vegetables or as a sandwich spread.

SERVES 6 (MAKES 2 CUPS)

> **2 cups spinach, well washed, stems removed, chopped**
> **One 10.5-ounce package firm silken tofu, drained**
> **1½ tablespoons lemon juice**
> **3 tablespoons chopped green onion**
> **½ teaspoon garlic powder**
> **½ teaspoon cumin**
> **2 tablespoons fresh savory**

Steam the spinach 2 to 3 minutes. In a food processor, puree all the ingredients until smooth. Chill for 2 to 4 hours. Serve as a dip with fresh vegetables or as a sandwich spread.

White Bean Red Pepper Spread

CHEF DEL SROUFE | WELLNESS FORUM FOODS

I LOVE HUMMUS, and there are plenty of good low-fat hummus recipes out there, but now and then I want something a little different. This spread is great as a dip for veggies or as a filling for sandwiches.

SERVES 4 TO 5

> **One 16-ounce can cannellini beans, drained and rinsed**
> **4 teaspoons mellow white miso**
> **1 roasted red bell pepper**
> **1 garlic clove, minced**
> **2 tablespoons fresh lemon juice**
> **Zest of 1 lemon**
> **Cayenne pepper**

Puree all the ingredients in the bowl of a food processor until smooth and creamy.

Eggplant Pecan Pesto

JO STEPANIAK | *BREAKING THE FOOD SEDUCTION* BY NEAL BARNARD, MD

HERE'S A SUPERB dairy-free pesto that is very simple to prepare. It is equally delicious as a dip or topping served at room temperature, or as a warm sauce over pasta or grains.

MAKES ABOUT 3 CUPS

½ **cup water**
1 **medium onion, diced**
½ **teaspoon crushed garlic**
1 **large eggplant, peeled**
1 **cup pecans**
½ **cup fresh basil, firmly packed**
2 **to 3 tablespoon fresh lemon juice**
2 **to 4 tablespoon light miso**

1. Heat water in a large nonstick skillet. Add onion and garlic and cook over medium-high heat for 5 minutes.
2. Meanwhile, cut eggplant into ½-inch cubes. Add to onion, cover, and reduce heat to medium. Cook, stirring often, until eggplant is very soft, about 25 to 30 minutes. If necessary, add a little more water to keep eggplant from sticking to pan.
3. When tender, transfer eggplant mixture to blender. Add remaining ingredients and process until completely smooth. Mixture will be thick.
4. Serve immediately while warm or at room temperature. Store leftovers in refrigerator and reheat to serve.

Arugula Pesto Risotto

MOIRA NORDHOLT | THE FEEL GOOD GURU

THIS DISH HAS a creaminess and stickiness reminiscent of the traditional Italian dish, without the butter, white wine, cheese, and beef stock. The pesto is a fresh, green-tasting version with arugula and spinach, ripe avocado instead of olive oil, and a generous blob of mild miso for a "cheesy" flavor. The avocado gives it a great creaminess that sticks nicely to the rice. Start with a pot of hot cooked, organic short-grain brown rice.

MAKES ENOUGH PESTO FOR 6 SERVINGS OF RICE

> 1 ripe avocado
> 4 cups organic arugula, loosely packed
> 4 cups organic spinach, loosely packed
> 1 small bunch of basil
> 1 small bunch of parsley
> 5 garlic cloves
> 3 tablespoons mild white miso
> ¼ cup unsalted vegetable broth
> ½ cup hemp seeds

1. Cut the avocados in half and discard their pits and peels. Puree the avocado, arugula, spinach, basil, parsley, garlic, miso, and vegetable broth in a food processor until creamy. Add hemp seeds and pulse to combine. If you like your pesto a little thinner, carefully add small amounts of water until it reaches your desired consistency.
2. Stir the pesto into warm brown rice and serve.

> **TIP ▶** You can use any leftover pesto to toss with penne noodles or any pasta, use as a delicious spread on toast, or dollop into carved zucchini or cucumber rounds for an elegant raw h'ors d'oeuvre.

VARIATIONS:

▶ Sprinkle with vegan "Parmesan": Pulse together about a cup of organic walnuts with half a cup of nutritional yeast and a teaspoon of Celtic sea salt.

▶ For a heartier risotto with some crunch, stir in kale ribbons, diced red pepper, and diced zucchini. For a little zing, add a squeeze of lemon.

Lettuce Wraps

LEANNE CAMPBELL DISLA | *WHOLE PLANTS COOKBOOK*

THE LETTUCE MAKES a crispy, light wrapping around the savory, flavorful filling. Children like to wrap their own, and you can make these larger or smaller depending on whether they're the appetizer or the main dish.

MAKES 6 TO 10 WRAPS

6 to 10 large butter lettuce leaves

¼ cup plus 2 tablespoons water

1 cup chopped water chestnuts

3 garlic cloves, minced

1 tablespoon diced fresh ginger

3 green onions, diced

2 large carrots, grated or thinly sliced

1 celery stalk, finely chopped

2 tablespoons sesame seeds

1 package (12 to 14 ounces) extra firm tofu, drained and cut into thin slices

2 tablespoons lime juice

2 tablespoons tamari

½ cup dry-roasted peanuts

Salt and black pepper

1. Wash the lettuce leaves, then pat dry and set aside. In a medium skillet, add ¼ cup of the water and the water chestnuts, garlic, ginger, green onions, carrots, and celery. Cook over medium-high heat until the onions are translucent. Add the remaining 2 tablespoons water and the sesame seeds, tofu, lime juice, and tamari. Cook for 1 to 2 minutes.
2. Remove the skillet from the heat and stir in the peanuts and season with salt and pepper.
3. Place 2 to 3 tablespoons of the mixture in the center of a whole lettuce leaf and fold the edges over the filling. Repeat with the remaining leaves and mixture. Enjoy.

Kalamata Olive Crostini

ANASTASIA ST. JOHN | COMPASSIONATE DIET AND LIFESTYLE ADVOCATE

THIS IS A quick and easy savory appetizer. Leftovers can be used as a sandwich spread.

SERVES 8

>   1 cup pitted kalamata olives
>   1 garlic clove
>   1 teaspoon dried rosemary
>   1 teaspoon dried oregano
>   Sprouted whole grain bread, sliced

1. Heat the oven to 450°F.
2. Puree the olives, garlic, and herbs in a food processor until they form a paste.
3. Cut the bread slices into quarters, place on a baking sheet, and lightly toast in the oven. Spread olive paste onto each piece, and serve.

Easy Quesadillas

ELISE MURPHY | T. COLIN CAMPBELL FOUNDATION

THESE QUESADILLAS ARE very simple to make. If you don't have time to make the "cheese" part of the recipe, you can use any type of hummus instead.

MAKES 10 QUESADILLAS

> **2 cups cooked chickpeas**
> **3 tablespoons nutritional yeast**
> **2 cloves garlic**
> **2 tablespoons tahini**
> **2 tablespoons white wine vinegar**
> **2 tablespoons light miso**
> **1 tablespoon low-sodium soy sauce**
> **1 teaspoon onion powder**
> **1 teaspoon cumin**
> **1 teaspoon salt**
> **1 teaspoon paprika**
> **½ teaspoon dried mustard**
> **Twenty 10-inch whole-wheat tortillas**
> **1 to 2 jars of your favorite salsa**
> **1 can vegan, oil-free, refried beans (I use La Preferida brand black beans)**
> **2 bunches scallions, chopped**
> **Additional salsa and guacamole for topping**

1. Combine the chickpeas, nutritional yeast, garlic, tahini, vinegar, miso, soy sauce, onion powder, cumin, salt, paprika, and mustard in the bowl of a food processor fitted with the "S" blade. Pulse until the ingredients become a smooth paste. You may have to scrape the sides down. Set aside. This is the "cheese."
2. Heat a large skillet over medium-high heat.
3. Spread a thin layer of the "cheese" on one tortilla. Top with a thin layer of refried beans, spread with a few spoonfuls of salsa, and sprinkle with scallions.
4. Top with a second tortilla and gently place in the heated skillet. Dry-fry for 3 to 5 minutes, until the tortilla is crispy and starting to brown on the bottom. Flip and cook the other side until crisp and browned.
5. Remove from the skillet and slice into wedges.
6. Repeat with the remaining tortillas.
7. Serve hot, topped with additional salsa or guacamole.

Yamadillas

MARY MCDOUGALL | THE MCDOUGALL PROGRAM

SERVE THESE WITH salsa (and guacamole, if you wish) spooned over the top. These can be eaten with a knife and fork or cut into wedges, picked up with your fingers, and dunked into the salsa and/or guacamole.

SERVES 8

2 pounds garnet yams, peeled and cut into chunks

2 tablespoons vegetable broth

2 tablespoons chopped green chiles

2 teaspoons lime juice

1 teaspoon minced chipotle in adobo sauce

¾ teaspoon ground cumin

½ teaspoon minced garlic

One 15-ounce can black beans, drained and rinsed

8 whole wheat tortillas

Fresh salsa of your choice

Guacamole (or Pea Guacamole, page 74)

1. Put the yams in a stainless-steel saucepot with enough water to cover. Bring to a boil, reduce heat, cover, and cook for about 12 minutes, until soft. Drain off the water and add the vegetable broth to the yams. Mash with a potato masher until quite smooth, then stir in the green chiles, lime juice, chipotle, cumin, and garlic. Mix well, stir in the black beans, and mix again.

2. Heat a nonstick griddle or large skillet over medium heat. Spread some of the yam mixture on half of a tortilla, then fold over and flatten. Place the folded tortilla on the griddle and cook for about 2½ minutes on each side, flipping several times to make sure it doesn't burn. Repeat with the remaining yam mixture and tortillas. Serve with salsa and/or guacamole spooned over the top.

TIP ▶ This makes quite a large amount. However, they store well overnight in the refrigerator and, reheated on the griddle the next day, they'll taste just like they were freshly made.

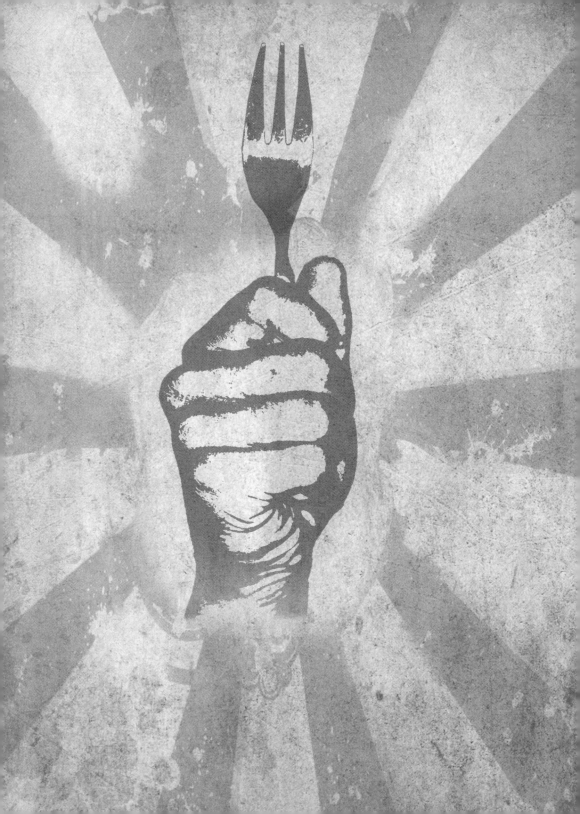

Acorn Squash Soup

ALAN GOLDHAMER AND DOUG LISLE | *THE HEALTH PROMOTING COOKBOOK*

THIS SMOOTH, VELVETY soup has a beautiful orange color and makes a nice presentation with a sprig of parsley as a garnish.

SERVES 8

> 7 cups vegetable stock or water
>
> 3 acorn squash, peeled and chopped
>
> 2 large carrots, peeled and chopped
>
> 1 large yam, peeled and chopped
>
> 1 teaspoon ground ginger
>
> 1 teaspoon sage
>
> 2 cups fresh or frozen corn kernels

1. In an 8-quart soup pot, bring the stock or water to a boil and stir in all the ingredients except the corn. Cook over medium-high heat for 20 minutes, or until the squash is soft.
2. Blend the soup in batches in a food processor or blender until smooth. Return to the pot, add the corn, and reheat on low for 10 minutes.

SOUPS

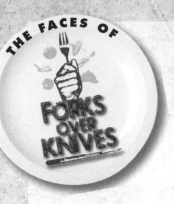

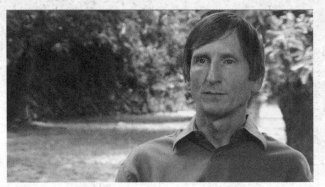

Doug Lisle, PhD

DR. DOUG LISLE, a graduate of the University of California at San Diego, received the President's Fellowship and was a DuPont Scholar at the University of Virginia, where he completed his doctor of philosophy in clinical psychology. The author of *The Pleasure Trap*, Doug has worked with Colin Campbell, John McDougall, and other scientists in analyzing the impact of dietary and lifestyle changes in the treatment of chronic disease.

Doug's career choices were highly influenced by his study of genetics, which motivated Doug to understand self-destructive behavior from a new viewpoint—that addictive habits are the result of our instincts chasing illusions (what he calls "pleasure traps"). Today, Doug's practice is devoted to helping clients understand how to master and overcome self-sabotage.

"The health problems we see today are being caused by dietary excess," he says. "People are simply eating too many calories. We don't need to debate about whether it is too much fat or too many carbohydrates—the truth is that it is too much food. And the question is: Why?

"What we often hear is that people have become too sedentary, or to overly indulgent. But those explanations don't stand up to scientific scrutiny—after all, there's no reason why we would suddenly be more indulgent, a *lot* more indulgent, than we were just twenty or thirty years ago. So it must be something else.

"That 'something else' is what I call *the pleasure trap*. It's what happens when our natural psychology—built for an ancient world where getting enough to eat was a struggle—collides with the modern environment, which is filled to the brim with excess.

"All complex animals have within them what we call the motivational triad: a three-part motivational guidance system that directs them to (1) seek out pleasure, (2) avoid pain, and (3) conserve energy. In the natural world, that meant finding the ripest foods, avoiding predators, and taking every available shortcut to save precious calories.

"This system is inside every creature from a grasshopper to a gazelle, and it moves human behavior as well. The problem is that if you are 'smart' enough, you can trick the system—that is, you can create materials and experiences that short-circuit this machinery, so that a choice *feels* right, but it *isn't*. Today we see the effects of these tricks everywhere, from using drugs to smoking cigarettes to drinking alcohol, but the most widely used trick of all is eating highly processed foods.

"The method is the same in each case. Drugs, alcohol, processed foods— they overstimulate the pleasure mechanism, and the result is behavior that is tipped out of balance and out of control. This is the pleasure trap, where the ancient message of pleasure tells us that we are doing the right thing. But we're not.

"The modern economy's ingenuity at doing this trick has gotten much more commanding in just the last few years. *That* is why we now have such astounding epidemics of obesity, heart disease, cancer, diabetes, and other problems today. These are diseases caused by an overly rich diet that beckons us to overindulge, again and again, unless we are fortunate enough to understand and avoid the pleasure trap."

Raw Dream of Tomato Soup

CHEF AJ | *UNPROCESSED*

A MUCH HEALTHIER version of a childhood favorite with a twist, reminiscent of Campbell's Cream of Tomato Soup.

SERVES 4 AS AN APPETIZER OR 2 AS AN ENTRÉE

> **1 pound Roma tomatoes, chopped**
> **2 red bell peppers, seeded**
> **1 garlic clove**
> **6 to 8 large fresh basil leaves**
> **Juice of 1 lemon**
> **2 tablespoons sun-dried tomato powder (see tip)**
> **¼ teaspoon chipotle powder (or more, to taste)**
> **½ cup shelled hemp seeds, optional**

Puree the tomatoes, bell peppers, basil, lemon juice, tomato powder, and chipotle powder in a high-powered blender until smooth. Add the hemp seeds and blend again until creamy. The high-powered blender will warm the soup without its being heated on the stove. Serve immediately.

TIP ▶ If you can't find sun-dried tomato powder you can easily make your own: Just grind hard sun-dried tomatoes (not oil-packed ones) in a coffee grinder.

Sunny Orange Yam Bisque

CHRISTY MORGAN | THE BLISSFUL CHEF

NOT ONLY CAN you make this soup in under 30 minutes, but it's gluten free, soy free, and full of antioxidants and beta carotene from the orange vegetables. The whole family will enjoy it!

SERVES 2 TO 3

> **3 cups water or broth**
> **1 cup peeled and cubed butternut squash**
> **3 cups peeled and cubed sweet potato**
> **1 teaspoon dried thyme**
> **¼ teaspoon nutmeg**
> **1 tablespoon nutritional yeast**
> **1 teaspoon apple cider vinegar**
> **Tamari**
> **Fresh herbs**

1. Bring water, squash, and a pinch of salt to a boil in a saucepan. Cover and simmer for 5 minutes. Add the sweet potato, thyme, and nutmeg and stir. Bring back to a boil, then lower the heat and simmer until all the veggies are tender, about 10 minutes. Let soup cool slightly.
2. Puree the soup in a blender until smooth. Return the soup to the saucepan, add the nutritional yeast and vinegar, stir, and cook for a few minutes until hot. Season with tamari as needed. Serve garnished with fresh herbs.

Yam and Split Pea Soup with Tarragon

ANN CRILE ESSELSTYN

THIS SOUP IS simple and so delicious with its subtle tarragon taste and the slightly sweet yams. It cooks in two stages so the peas become creamy and the yams and onions keep their texture. If available, use garnet yams, which are a deeper color and sweeter than jewel yams or the pale-yellow sweet potatoes. (Don't bother peeling them.) Fresh tarragon makes all the difference.

This makes a great lunch, or serve it for dinner with a wonderful green salad and bread or toasted pita.

SERVES 6 TO 8

8 cups (2 quarts) vegetable broth or water
2 cups split green peas
1 bay leaf
½ teaspoon dry mustard
1 large red onion, chopped (about 2 cups)
3 medium yams, diced (7 to 8 cups)
½ cup chopped fresh tarragon (about a ¾-ounce container) or 2 teaspoons dried
Black pepper

Put the broth or water, split peas, bay leaf, and mustard into a soup pot. Bring to a boil, then lower heat, cover, and simmer 40 minutes, or until the peas begin to break down. Add the red onion, yams, and tarragon and stir. Simmer for 30 minutes, or until the yams are tender and the peas are creamy.

Split Pea Soup

MATT LEDERMAN AND ALONA PULDE—WITH THANKS TO SHOSHANA PULDE | *KEEP IT SIMPLE, KEEP IT WHOLE*

IT'S GRATIFYING THAT something so simple to make has such good flavor. We like to eat this with a green salad for an easy, healthy meal.

SERVES 4

- **1 onion, chopped**
- **1½ cups split peas**
- **2 large carrots, shredded**
- **10 cups boiling water**
- **2 tablespoons vegan chicken-soup-style vegetable powder**
- **Salt and black pepper, optional**
- **Fresh parsley, optional**

Sauté the onion in a large soup pot with a little water until yellow. Add the split peas, carrots, and water and bring to a boil. Add the chicken-soup-style powder and reduce the heat. Simmer for about an hour, stirring periodically to prevent sticking. Add salt and pepper to taste. Serve warm, garnished with a little chopped parsley.

Chilled Avocado Soup

TAL RONNEN | *QUANTUM WELLNESS* BY KATHY FRESTON

ON WARM-WEATHER DAYS a cup of this chilled soup makes for a jolt of green goodness—and the perfect start to lunch or dinner.

SERVES 4

- **2 ripe avocados, halved and pitted**
- **⅓ cup peas, cooked and cooled**
- **4 cups cold vegetable stock**
- **Juice from 1 lime**
- **Salt and pepper to taste**

Puree the ingredients in a blender until smooth.

Yellow Split Pea and Leek Soup

LEWIS FREEDMAN AND PRISCILLA TIMBERLAKE | *COMMUNITY DINNERS SERVED WITH LOVE*

THIS TASTY, SIMPLE soup takes very little preparation time and is still very rich and satisfying.

SERVES 8

> 2 cups yellow split peas
>
> 6 cups water
>
> 2 carrots, cut into small dice
>
> 1 red onion, cut into small dice
>
> 3 leeks, white and green parts separated, diced small
>
> 4 celery stalks, cut into small dice
>
> ½ teaspoon sea salt
>
> 2 tablespoons tamari

1. Bring 6 cups of water to a boil and add the peas. Reduce the heat to medium-low and cook until the peas are soft, about 2 hours.
2. When the peas are soft, add carrots, onion, and white parts of the leeks. Cook for 20 to 30 minutes until the vegetables are soft. Add celery and cook for 5 minutes. Add salt, tamari, and the green part of the leeks and cook for 7 to 10 minutes more. Serve.

Cream of Broccoli Deluxe

ANASTASIA ST. JOHN | COMPASSIONATE DIET AND LIFESTYLE ADVOCATE

THIS SOUP IS very hearty . . . perfect as a meal in itself. A large pot of this rich and creamy soup won't last long!

SERVES 6

> **6 cups vegetable stock or boullion**
> **1 rounded cup raw cashews**
> **1 medium onion, finely chopped**
> **1 celery stalk, finely chopped**
> **1 large carrot, chopped**
> **1 garlic clove, minced**
> **½ large red bell pepper, chopped**
> **2 medium unpeeled potatoes, cubed**
> **1 large head broccoli, including stem, chopped (about 4 cups)**
> **2 teaspoons dried thyme**
> **1 teaspoon sea salt**
> **½ teaspoon black pepper**

1. Puree 1 cup of the vegetable stock with the cashews in a blender until smooth. Set aside.
2. In a large pot, cook the onion, celery, and carrot over medium heat in 1 cup of the vegetable stock for 5 minutes. Add the garlic, bell pepper, and potatoes and cook for 2 more minutes. Add the remaining 4 cups of vegetable stock and the broccoli, thyme, salt, and black pepper, and bring to a boil over high heat. Cover and simmer until the broccoli and potatoes are soft, about 10 minutes.
3. Add the cashew mixture to the soup and stir until mixed. Remove the pot from heat and puree about half the soup, in small batches, until smooth. Return pureed soup to the pot and reheat, stirring well. Serve.

Bean and Barley Chowder

JO STEPANIAK | *BREAKING THE FOOD SEDUCTION* BY NEAL BARNARD, MD

BARLEY IS DELICIOUS, not to mention an excellent course of soluble fiber, which reduces blood cholesterol levels. The longer you cook this thick and hearty soup, the creamier and richer tasting it becomes.

MAKES ABOUT 2 QUARTS

8 cups water or vegetable stock
1 cup dry baby lima beans, soaked overnight and drained
1 cup chopped onion
1 cup chopped carrot
1 celery stalk, finely chopped
½ cup pearl barley
1 tablespoon crushed garlic
1 teaspoon thyme
Salt and pepper

Place water and beans in a large soup pot and bring to a boil. Add remaining ingredients, except salt and pepper. Return to a boil, reduce heat to medium, cover, and simmer until barley and beans are tender and broth is creamy, about 1½ to 2 hours. Season with salt and pepper to taste. Serve hot.

Creamy Corn Chowder

CHEF AJ | *UNPROCESSED*

I PREFER THIS soup served cold like a gazpacho.

SERVES 4 AS AN APPETIZER OR 2 AS AN ENTRÉE

- 2½ cups plain, unsweetened almond milk, chilled
- 2½ cups fresh or frozen organic corn kernels (thawed), plus more for optional garnish
- 1 small shallot
- 1 ripe avocado, plus more for optional garnish
- Scallions or fresh cilantro, optional

Puree all ingredients in a blender until smooth. Ladle into bowls and sprinkle with scallions, diced avocado, and corn kernels.

VARIATION:

► For even more flavor, add some sun-dried tomato powder and chipotle powder.

Zingy Italian White Bean Soup

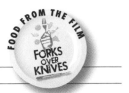

MOIRA NORDHOLT | THE FEEL GOOD GURU

THIS RECIPE BEGINS the night before, when you will need to wash your dried cannellini beans and cover them in water to soak. Start cooking them a little while before you begin chopping vegetables, and they should be ready by the time you're ready to make your soup.

SERVES 2 GENEROUSLY

1 cup dried cannellini beans (white Italian kidney beans), soaked

1 unsalted vegetable bouillon cube

4 garlic cloves, minced

Half a red onion, diced

2 stalks celery, diced

3 stalks fresh fennel, or half a fennel bulb, diced

1 zucchini, diced

1 bunch of fresh spinach, chopped

1 teaspoon oregano

4 fresh sage leaves, chopped

1 teaspoon parsley

Splash tamari

1 teaspoon sea salt

Freshly ground black pepper

1 lemon

1. Drain the beans, then put them in a pot, cover with water, and bring to a boil. Lower the heat and simmer until al dente.
2. In a large soup pot, dissolve the bouillon cube in ¼ cup water over medium heat. Add garlic and onion. Cook, stirring constantly, until they sweat. Add celery and fennel with a pinch of sea salt. Allow the vegetables to heat through and soften. Cover the vegetables with spring water and bring to a boil. Simmer for 5 or 10 minutes.
3. Add zucchini, spinach, cooked beans, oregano, sage, parsley, tamari, sea salt, and black pepper. Simmer for another 5 minutes, or until the zucchini is cooked but not mushy. Turn off the heat. Squeeze the juice of a whole lemon into the soup. Adjust the seasonings to your liking and serve.

Lentil Soup

CHEF DEL SROUFE | WELLNESS FORUM FOODS

LENTILS, A SMALL but nutritionally mighty member of the legume family, are a very good source of cholesterol-lowering fiber. They are quick and easy to prepare and readily absorb a variety of flavors from other foods and seasonings.

SERVES 6

> 1 large onion, finely diced
> 2 medium carrots, finely diced
> 2 celery stalks, finely diced
> 3 garlic cloves, minced
> 3 tablespoons tomato paste
> 2 bay leaves
> 1 teaspoon fresh thyme, minced
> 1 teaspoon fresh tarragon, minced
> ¼ bunch of fresh parsley, finely chopped
> 1½ cups green lentils
> 2 quarts vegetable stock
> 1½ teaspoons sea salt
> 2 tablespoons Dijon mustard
> Black pepper

1. Sauté the onion, carrot, and celery in a large soup pot over medium-high heat for 7 to 8 minutes. If necessary, add 1 to 2 tablespoons of water at a time to keep the vegetables from sticking to the pan.
2. Add the garlic, tomato paste, bay leaves, thyme, tarragon, and parsley. Cook for another minute. Add the lentils, vegetable stock, and sea salt. Bring to a boil, then lower the heat and simmer, partially covered, until the lentils are tender, 25 to 35 minutes. Stir in the mustard and season with black pepper. Remove the bay leaves before serving.

Red Lentil Soup

DARSHANA THACKER | AYURVEDIC VEGAN CHEF

THE LENTILS AND grain combination make this a hearty one-dish meal. You can substitute the vegetables below with other vegetables of your choice. If you're using barley instead of brown rice, you'll need to start soaking the barley a few hours before.

SERVES 4 TO 6

¼ cup barley or brown rice

4¾ cups water

1 cup red lentils

½ teaspoon cumin seeds

¼ cup finely chopped onion

¼ teaspoon green chile paste

½ teaspoon grated ginger

¼ cup finely chopped tomato

¼ teaspoon minced garlic

¼ teaspoon turmeric

¼ teaspoon salt

⅛ teaspoon black pepper

¼ cup cauliflower, cut into small florets

¼ cup carrot, cut into small pieces

¼ cup green beans, cut into small pieces

2 tablespoons lemon juice

1 tablespoon finely chopped fresh cilantro

1. If using barley, cover the barley with water and soak for 3 to 4 hours. Rinse thoroughly. Put barley and 1½ cups of the water into a pot and bring to a boil, then lower the heat and simmer until tender, about 15 to 20 minutes. Set aside.

2. If using brown rice, wash the rice and put into a pot with 1½ cups of the water. Bring to a boil, reduce the heat, and simmer for about 5 minutes, then cover and cook for 10 to 15 minutes. Set aside.

3. Wash the lentils thoroughly, then put into a soup pot with 3 cups of the water and bring to a boil. Lower the heat and cook until tender.

4. Lightly roast the cumin seeds in a sauté pan, 1 to 2 minutes. Add the onion, chile paste, and ginger, and cook for a minute, stirring constantly, then add ¼ cup of the water. Cook until the onion is translucent,

3 to 4 minutes. Add the tomato, garlic, turmeric, salt, and black pepper and cook until the tomato softens, about 5 minutes.

5. Add the tomato mixture and the cauliflower, carrot, and green beans to the lentils. Bring to a boil, then lower the heat and simmer until the vegetables are soft, about 15 minutes. Add the cooked rice or barley and bring the soup to a boil. Add the lemon juice and serve hot, garnished with the cilantro.

Hearty Dal Soup

MARY MCDOUGALL | THE MCDOUGALL PROGRAM

THIS IS ONE of our favorite soups. I make this at least once a week.

SERVES 4

> 3 ¼ cups water
> 1 onion, chopped
> 2 garlic cloves, crushed
> 1½ teaspoons grated fresh ginger
> 1 teaspoon smoked paprika
> ¼ teaspoon ground cumin
> Freshly ground black pepper
> 1 cup dried red lentils
> One 15-ounce can chickpeas, drained and rinsed
> One 14½-ounce can diced tomatoes
> 2 cups chunked Yukon Gold potatoes
> 1 tablespoon lemon juice
> 1 to 2 teaspoons chile paste (sambal oelek)
> 2 cups chopped chard
> Sea salt, optional

1. Heat ¼ cup of the water in a large soup pot over medium-high heat. Add the onion and garlic and cook, stirring occasionally, for 3 to 4 minutes until softened.

2. Add the ginger, paprika, cumin, and black pepper to the pot and stir well. Add the remaining 3 cups water and the lentils, chickpeas, tomatoes, and potatoes. Bring to a boil, reduce heat, cover, and simmer for 50 minutes, or until lentils are tender. Add lemon juice, chile paste (start with 1 teaspoon and add more to taste), and chard. Cook for 5 to 7 more minutes, until chard is tender. Season with a bit of sea salt, if desired. Serve hot.

Exsalus's Black Bean Soup

MATT LEDERMAN AND ALONA PULDE | *KEEP IT SIMPLE, KEEP IT WHOLE*

TRY THIS HEARTY soup for a delicious meal, with a little bit of a kick from the peppers.

SERVES 4

> **1½ cup chopped onions**
> **1 cup chopped carrots**
> **1 cup chopped celery**
> **Six 15-ounce cans black beans**
> **1 pound frozen corn**
> **Four 16-ounce cans crushed tomatoes spiced with green chiles**
> **2 banana peppers, chopped**
> **1 jalapeño pepper, chopped**
> **3 bunches of greens (such as kale, collards, or chard), chopped or torn,**
> **with stems removed**
> **½ to 1 cup fresh cilantro**
> **Oil-free corn chips**

1. Put 1 cup of the onions and the carrots, celery, black beans, corn, tomatoes, banana peppers, and jalepenos into a large soup pot. Bring to a boil, then reduce the heat and simmer for 30 minutes.
2. While the soup is cooking, sauté the remaining ½ cup onions and the kale, collards, and chard in a saucepan with a little vegetable broth or water for about 10 minutes.
3. Puree the cooked greens and fresh cilantro in a food processor. Add blended greens to the soup and stir well. Serve with crushed-up corn chips mixed in.

Nutrient-Rich Smoky Black Bean Soup

CHEF AJ | *UNPROCESSED*

THE MEXICAN OREGANO called for in this recipe is bolder than typical oregano, in aroma as well as in texture. The aroma is said to stand up better to the hearty flavors often used in Mexican dishes, and has a distinct, pleasing citrus note. If you can't find it, regular oregano is fine.

No one will guess that there are two pounds of greens hidden in this delicious soup. And because it will be pureed, there is no need to cut anything up. This recipe makes enough for a party!

SERVES 30

> **12 cups (3 quarts) low-sodium vegetable broth**
> **Six 15-ounce cans salt-free black beans**
> **2 red onions, peeled**
> **8 garlic cloves, peeled**
> **1 pound cremini mushrooms**
> **1 pound baby bok choy (about 3 stalks)**
> **1 pound greens (kale, collard, mustard, chard, or a combination), chopped**
> **2 large sweet potatoes, peeled**
> **Two 16-ounce bags frozen corn, defrosted**
> **2 tablespoons sun-dried tomato powder**
> **2 tablespoons ground cumin**
> **2 tablespoons Mexican oregano**
> **1 tablespoon chipotle paste or ¼ teaspoon chipotle powder**
> **Juice and zest of 4 limes**
> **Pepitas, optional**
> **Fresh cilantro, optional**

1. Pour the broth into a large soup pot and bring to a boil. Reduce the heat and add the beans, onions, garlic, mushrooms, bok choy, greens, and sweet potatoes; stir. Simmer uncovered for 30 minutes.
2. Remove the soup from the heat and blend with an immersion blender. Stir in the corn, sun-dried tomato powder, cumin, oregano, chipotle paste, and lime juice. Add more chipotle paste to taste and garnish with pepitas and cilantro, if desired.

TIP ▶ If you can't get salt-free canned beans, be sure to drain your beans and then rinse them thoroughly before using.

TIP ▶ If you do not have a handheld immersion blender, you can carefully blend the unseasoned soup in small batches in a regular blender, then return it to the pot before stirring in the remaining ingredients.

TIP ▶ Chipotle paste, which gives this soup an authentic flavor, is available at Whole Foods Market and online at www.shop.chipotlepeople.com. It has only 10 milligrams of sodium per teaspoon and is a wonderful addition to chili, guacamole, and salsa. If you can't find it, you can substitute one to three canned chipotle chiles, which are readily available in the international foods section of most supermarkets. *Muy sabrosa!*

Hearty Minestrone Soup

MARY MCDOUGALL | THE MCDOUGALL PROGRAM

THIS IS A quicker version of our favorite minestrone soup that uses canned beans instead of the dried kidney beans. All of the delicious flavor is still here, though, and with a loaf of fresh bread it makes a hearty meal for several people.

SERVES 6 TO 8

1 onion, chopped

2 celery stalks, sliced

2 carrots, sliced

1 teaspoon crushed garlic

6 cups vegetable broth

½ cup chopped green beans

1½ cups chunked potatoes

1½ cups shredded cabbage

One 14½-ounce can chopped tomatoes

One 8-ounce can tomato sauce

One 15-ounce can chickpeas, drained and rinsed

One 15-ounce can cannellini beans, drained and rinsed

¼ cup parsley

1½ teaspoons basil

Freshly ground black pepper

½ cup uncooked whole wheat or brown rice pasta

1. Put the onion, celery, carrots, and garlic in a large pot with ¼ cup of the vegetable broth. Cook over medium-high heat, stirring occasionally, for 2 to 3 minutes, until vegetables soften slightly.
2. Add the remaining 5¾ cups broth and the green beans, potatoes, cabbage, tomatoes, tomato sauce, chickpeas, cannellini beans, parsley, basil, and black pepper to the pot. Bring to a boil, then reduce the heat, cover, and cook for 45 minutes.
3. Add the pasta, stir well, and continue to cook for another 15 minutes, or until the pasta is tender.

The Quickest Black Bean Salad

ANN CRILE ESSELSTYN | *PREVENT AND REVERSE HEART DISEASE*

WE COULD EAT this for every meal in summer, even breakfast. It is the salad I make when I have to take a dish to an event because it is so quick to make, everyone comes back for seconds, and it is the best advertisement for delicious NO OIL eating. It is easy to expand by adding more tomatoes or frozen corn.

SERVES 4

> Two 16-ounce cans black beans drained and rinsed WELL!
> 1 very large tomato, chopped
> 1 package frozen corn
> ½ Vidalia onion, chopped
> 1 can sliced water chestnuts, drained and rinsed
> 1 bunch cilantro, chopped
> ½ lime, juice and zest
> 3 tablespoons balsamic vinegar or more to taste

1. Add beans, tomatoes, corn, onion, and water chestnuts to a bowl (glass looks pretty) and mix. Rinsing the beans well keeps the salad from looking gray.
2. Add cilantro, lime, and balsamic vinegar and mix again. Serve alone or with cucumber open-faced sandwiches for a perfect meal.

Garbanzo Spinach Salad

MARY MCDOUGALL | THE MCDOUGALL PROGRAM

THIS IS ONE of my favorite salads, and very often I eat this right after putting it together. It keeps well in the refrigerator for several days.

SERVES 4 TO 6

Three 15-ounce cans chickpeas, drained and rinsed
2 cups loosely packed chopped fresh spinach
½ cup chopped red bell pepper
½ cup chopped yellow bell pepper
3 green onions, finely chopped
½ cup oil-free dressing
Freshly ground black pepper

Combine the beans and the spinach, bell peppers, and green onions in a bowl. Pour the dressing over and toss to mix. Season with black pepper. Refrigerate for 1 to 2 hours for best flavor.

Woodstock Peace Salad with Tahini Dressing

KRIS CARR | *CRAZY SEXY DIET*

IT'S UP TO you what to put into this salad—take your pick from the ingredients I suggest below.

SALAD

Organic mixed greens (romaine, arugula, or spinach)
Diced cucumbers
Red peppers
Shredded carrots
Broccoli florets
Diced red onions
Shredded purple cabbage
Sprouts of your choice (my favorites are sunflower and mung bean sprouts)
Avocado
Olives
Hemp seeds

TAHINI DRESSING

1 cup tahini
½ cup lemon juice
1 garlic clove
Purified water (use enough to thin out and create the desired consistency)
Salt and pepper to taste

1. Prepare the salad ingredients of your choice and toss them together.
2. Whisk together all the dressing ingredients in a bowl until combined.
3. Dress the salad and serve.

Coleslaw

KAREN CAMPBELL | THE CAMPBELL FAMILY

THIS REFRESHING SALAD will spice up any party or cookout.

SERVES 3

> 3 cups finely chopped cabbage
>
> 1 carrot, finely chopped
>
> 3 tablespoons vinegar
>
> 1 tablespoon sweetener, such as agave
>
> 2 tablespoons plant-based milk (see page 68)
>
> 1 tablespoon fat-free Nayonaise (soy dressing found in health food stores)
>
> ½ teaspoon dill
>
> ¼ teaspoon sea salt
>
> Black pepper

Put the vinegar, sweetener, milk, Nayonaise, dill, and salt into a bowl and stir well to combine. Add the cabbage and carrots and toss to mix. Sprinkle with black pepper to taste.

Mango-Lime Bean Salad

ANN CRILE ESSELSTYN | *PREVENT AND REVERSE HEART DISEASE*

EVERYONE LOVES THIS, so make double or even triple the recipe. It VANISHES in a flash! It really is our all-time favorite summer salad. The red onion adds a dash of color, and the zest (the peel) intensifies the lime flavor. Make sure there is PLENTY of lime—it makes the difference!

SERVES 2

> 1 mango, peeled and diced
>
> One 15-ounce can cannellini beans, drained and rinsed
>
> Red onion, diced, to taste (start with ½)
>
> Cilantro . . . a lot (½ cup or more!)
>
> Zest of 1 lime
>
> Juice of 1 juicy lime, squeezed (2 tablespoons or to taste)

Combine all ingredients and serve on a bed of arugala or baby lettuce or, best of all, mâche if you can find it. This is also good as a salsa.

Sweet Carrot Salad

ALAN GOLDHAMER AND DOUG LISLE | *THE HEALTH PROMOTING COOKBOOK*

A LIGHTER DISH reminiscent of Waldorf salad without the heavy sauce.

SERVES 3

6 carrots, thinly sliced
2 apples, peeled and diced
1 tablespoon apple juice
Juice of 1 lemon
½ teaspoon cinnamon
½ cup raisins

Steam the carrots for 5 minutes. Mix all the ingredients in a medium bowl. Chill the salad for 1 hour before serving.

Quinoa Salad with Currants

CHEF AJ | *UNPROCESSED*

THIS QUICK AND easy salad has the perfect blend of sweet and savory. Try red quinoa for a colorful change of pace.

SERVES 16

One 16-ounce box of quinoa
1 cup freshly squeezed lime juice (about 8 limes) and zest from limes
½ cup finely chopped scallions
½ cup finely chopped Italian parsley
½ cup finely chopped mint
2 cups currants
1 cup pomegranate seeds (when in season), optional

1. Prepare quinoa according to the directions on the package. Place in large bowl and allow to cool.
2. Pour over the lime juice over the quinoa. Add the lime zest, scallions, parsley, mint, currants, and pomegranate seeds and mix well. Chill.

Quinoa Garden Salad

MARY MCDOUGALL | THE MCDOUGALL PROGRAM

THIS SALAD IS bright and citrusy and full of flavor. It also contains two of my favorite ingredients, garbanzos and quinoa, so I make this often and enjoy it for lunch.

SERVES 6 TO 8

> 2 cups water
> 1 cup quinoa, well rinsed
> 1 red bell pepper, chopped
> 1 green bell pepper, chopped
> ½ yellow bell pepper, chopped
> 2 tomatoes, chopped
> 1 bunch of chopped green onions
> One 14½-ounce can chickpeas, drained and rinsed
> ½ cup chopped fresh parsley
> ¼ cup chopped fresh mint
> ½ cup fresh lemon juice
> 1 tablespoon soy sauce
> Tabasco sauce
> Freshly ground black pepper

1. Put the water and quinoa into a saucepan. Bring to a boil, reduce the heat, cover, and cook for 15 minutes, until water is absorbed. Remove from the heat and set aside.
2. Meanwhile, combine the bell peppers, tomatoes, green onions, beans, parsley, and mint in a large bowl. Add the cooked quinoa and mix well. Add the lemon juice, soy sauce, and several dashes of Tabasco sauce, and toss well to mix. Add black pepper to taste. Cover and refrigerate for at least 2 hours before serving.

TIP ▶ Quinoa can be very bitter unless it is rinsed well before cooking.

VARIATION:
▶ Use any combination of bell peppers—you need about 2½ cups total.

Mediterranean Quinoa Salad

MOIRA NORDHOLT | THE FEEL GOOD GURU

QUINOA WAS THE "gold of the Incas" because of the protein and energy it supplied their warriors. Yes, if you've got quinoa in your pantry, you're wealthy. This superfood is actually a seed, but cooks up quickly like a grain and has a really nice sort of creamy, mildly nutty flavor. I love cooking with quinoa, not just for its wonderful aroma and texture, but for its quick cooking time. You can whip up a pot in about 15 minutes.

SERVES 2 AS AN ENTRÉE OR 4 AS A SIDE

> 1½ cups quinoa
> 3 cups water
> ½ cup cooked organic chickpeas (or half a 15-ounce can of organic chickpeas)
> 5 sun-dried tomatoes, chopped
> ½ cup hulled hemp seeds
> ½ Persian or English cucumber, diced
> 2 tablespoons capers
> 3 large spicy olives, pitted and chopped
> ½ cup pine nuts, toasted
> Juice of 1 organic lemon
> Pink Himalayan sea salt

1. To cook the quinoa, rinse well, then cover with the 3 cups water; bring to a boil, then reduce the heat, cover, and cook for 15 minutes.
2. Put the chickpeas, tomatoes, hemp seeds, cucumber, capers, olives, and pine nuts into a bowl and mix well. Drizzle with lemon juice and add salt to taste. Depending how juicy your lemon is, you may wish to add more. You can serve this warm, chilled, or room temperature.

TIP▶ To make a batch of cooked chickpeas, first soak 1 cup dried chickpeas overnight in plenty of water. Drain, then put them in a saucepan and cover with 2 quarts of water. Bring to a boil, then reduce the heat and simmer until tender, about 1 to 2 hours.

VARIATION:
> ▶ Add the juice from an orange for a lovely sweet-and-tangy flavor.

Goddess Niçoise

ISA CHANDRA MOSKOWITZ | *APPETITE FOR REDUCTION*

SALADE NIÇOISE IS a bistro staple. It's steamed potatoes, crisp green beans, and salty Niçoise olives dunked in a lush dressing. Traditionally it is served with tuna, but I serve it with lightly mashed chickpeas that are spiked with briny capers. NYC sidewalk cafés are lined with ladies talking on their cell phones, reading French *Vogue*, and eating this salad. Now you can bring it home, sans all the bus exhaust in your face and the crazy drunk guy trying to steal the bread basket off your table.

Green Goddess Garlic Dressing is a perfect accompaniment, but you can also serve it with a more traditional balsamic vinaigrette if you prefer. Tiny red potatoes work best here, but if you can't find any, then chop up regular ones into 1-inch pieces. This recipe does make a bunch of dirty dishes, but be a goddess and have someone else clean them up! For time-management purposes, prepare the dressing while the potatoes are steaming, or (even better) prepare the dressing a day in advance.

SERVES 4

> One 16-ounce can chickpeas, drained and rinsed
> 2 tablespoons capers
> ½ pound small, whole red potatoes
> ½ pound green beans, stems removed
> ½ small red onion, cut into thin strips
> ⅓ cup Niçoise olives (kalamata olives work, too)
> 8 cups chopped red leaf lettuce
> 1 cup cherry tomatoes (orange ones if you can get them)
> Fresh parsley and chopped chives, for garnish
> About ¾ cup Green Goddess Garlic Dressing (page 114)

1. Prepare your steamer for the potatoes. Once it's ready, steam the potatoes for 10 to 15 minutes; they should be pierced easily with a fork. Meanwhile, prepare an ice bath by filling a mixing bowl halfway with ice water. Add the green beans to the steamer and steam for 2 more minutes, until the beans are bright green.
2. Transfer the potatoes and green beans to the ice bath immediately. Let them cool while you prepare everything else.
3. Place the chickpeas in a mixing bowl and use a small potato masher or a fork to mash them. There should be no whole chickpeas left, but they shouldn't be completely smooth like hummus, either; you want some

texture. Add the capers and 2 tablespoons of the dressing. Mix well and set aside.

4. To assemble, place the lettuce in wide bowls. In a Salade Niçoise, usually all the components are kept together, instead of tossed. Place a handful each of potatoes and green beans in piles on the lettuce, along with a wedge of sliced onion and a handful of tomatoes. Place a scoop of the chickpea mixture in the center and top with the olives. Garnish with fresh herbs and serve with the dressing on the side.

TIP ▶ This salad doesn't call for the entire recipe of the goddess dressing; reserve the rest for sandwiches the next day.

Green Goddess Garlic Dressing

ISA CHANDRA MOSKOWITZ | *APPETITE FOR REDUCTION*

THIS IS THE stuff! I don't use the word *mouthwatering* lightly, but the moment this dressing touches my tongue it just permeates every taste bud, and perhaps even the very core of my being. Herby, garlicky, tangy, luscious, vibrant . . . I'm gonna burn out all my food adjectives if I go on. I love to pour it on grain and bean salads. The tahini makes it a natural player in a Middle Eastern spread, and the miso makes it equally at home with Japanese dishes. But really, with all the flavors going on, it's kind of everyone's best friend. Again, use whichever miso you have on hand.

SERVES 6 (3 TABLESPOONS EACH)

2 to 3 average-size garlic cloves
½ cup fresh chives
½ cup fresh parsley
2 tablespoons tahini
2 tablespoons nutritional yeast
1 tablespoon miso
⅓ cup water
2 tablespoons freshly squeezed lemon juice
½ teaspoon salt

1. Pulse 2 cloves of garlic, the chives, and the parsley in a food processor just to chop everything up. Add the remaining ingredients and blend until very smooth. Use a rubber spatula to scrape down the sides a few times. Now you should adjust it to your liking. See if it needs more salt and garlic, and thin the dressing with a tablespoon or two of water, if needed. Note that it will thicken a bit as it's refrigerated, so if it appears thin, don't worry!
2. Transfer to a tightly sealed container and chill until ready to serve.

Romaine Salad with Fresh Strawberries and Strawberry Tarragon Dressing

CHEF DEL SROUFE | WELLNESS FORUM FOODS

MAKE THIS SALAD with the freshest strawberries when you can. It makes all the difference in the world! If you'd like, serve the salad with the dressing on the side so each guest can add as much or as little as they would like. The dressing really proves the point that you don't need to use oil to achieve a full flavor!

SERVES 4 AND MAKES ENOUGH DRESSING FOR 12

SALAD
1 large head of romaine lettuce, washed, dried, and cut into 1-inch pieces
1 medium red onion, thinly sliced
½ cup toasted sunflower seeds, optional
1 large carrot, peeled and grated
1 pint fresh strawberries, washed, hulled, and cut in half

DRESSING
4 cups strawberries, washed, hulled, and sliced
1 medium shallot, minced
½ cup balsamic vinegar
½ teaspoon freshly ground white pepper
½ cup agave nectar or brown rice syrup
1 tablespoon dried tarragon
1 teaspoon salt

1. Mix all the salad ingredients together in a large bowl.
2. Puree all the dressing ingredients in a blender until smooth and creamy, stopping once or twice to scrape down the sides.
3. Toss the salad with Strawberry Tarragon Dressing to taste.

Raspberry-Hemp Mixed Green Salad

ANASTASIA ST. JOHN | COMPASSIONATE DIET AND LIFESTYLE ADVOCATE

THIS SLIGHTLY SWEET salad is fresh and light.

SERVES 4

> **5 ounces mixed greens**
> **1 cup fresh or frozen raspberries, thawed**
> **1 medium carrot, shredded**
> **2 tablespoons hemp seeds**
> **Raspberry-Orange Vinaigrette dressing (recipe follows)**

Toss all the ingredients with Raspberry-Orange Vinaigrette dressing.

Raspberry-Orange Vinaigrette

ANASTASIA ST. JOHN | COMPASSIONATE DIET AND LIFESTYLE ADVOCATE

THIS DRESSING IS the perfect topping to the Raspberry-Hemp Mixed Green Salad or any summer salad.

> **1 cup orange juice**
> **½ cup fresh or frozen raspberries, thawed**
> **¼ cup balsamic vinegar**
> **Freshly ground black pepper**

Puree orange juice, raspberries, and balsamic vinegar in a blender until smooth. Add black pepper to taste.

Asian Salad Dressing

MARY MCDOUGALL | THE MCDOUGALL PROGRAM

A SIMPLE, YET fantastic, dressing that is usually in my refrigerator to dress many varieties of greens.

MAKES 1 CUP

⅓ **cup water**
¼ **cup rice vinegar**
¼ **cup low-sodium soy sauce**
½ **teaspoon red pepper flakes, optional**
¼ **teaspoon minced garlic**
¼ **teaspoon grated ginger**
¼ **teaspoon guar gum**

Combine all the ingredients in a small jar with a lid and shake until well mixed.

TIP ▶ Guar gum is a thickening agent that does not require cooking. It gives oil-free dressings a nice consistency for clinging to salad leaves.

Lemon-Ginger Salad Dressing

MOIRA NORDHOLT | THE FEEL GOOD GURU

YOUR BABY GREENS will sing with this simple and delicious salad dressing. Make it in advance and let it sit, covered, at room temperature until you're ready to serve. Fresh lemon and ginger go so nicely together, with just a touch of sweetness from the pure maple syrup. This recipe makes two salad portions.

SERVES 2

1-inch piece of fresh ginger, grated finely
Juice of 1 juicy lemon
2 tablespoons maple syrup

Mix all the ingredients together in a small bowl.

Jane's 3, 2, 1 Salad Dressing

ANN CRILE ESSELSTYN | *PREVENT AND REVERSE HEART DISEASE*

EVERY TIME WE eat our daughter Jane's salads we ask, "What is this delicious dressing?" It is easy to make and to adjust to personal taste.

MAKES ABOUT ⅓ CUP

> **3 tablespoons balsamic vinegar**
> **2 tablespoons mustard of choice**
> **1 tablespoon maple syrup**

Mix all ingredients in a small bowl with a whisk until smooth.

Citrus Chile Dressing

MARY MCDOUGALL | THE MCDOUGALL PROGRAM

A SPICY CITRUS dressing that really perks up your salads.

MAKES ABOUT 1½ CUPS

> **1 cup orange juice**
> **¼ cup Dijon mustard**
> **½ cup rice vinegar**
> **2 garlic cloves**
> **1 tablespoon chile powder**
> **1 tablespoon sweet chile sauce**
> **½ teaspoon guar gum**

Puree all the ingredients in a blender until smooth.

Avocado Dressing

LEANNE CAMPBELL DISLA | *WHOLE PLANTS COOKBOOK*

THIS DRESSING GIVES a tangy, Southwestern flavor. It works well on bean salads in addition to green ones.

SERVES 8

> **2 garlic cloves, minced**
> **¾ cup soft avocado**
> **¼ cup white wine**
> **2 tablespoons lime juice**
> **1 teaspoon Dijon mustard**
> **¼ teaspoon sea salt**
> **¼ teaspoon black pepper**

Put all the ingredients in the bowl of a food processor and pulse until well combined. Refrigerate overnight to blend the flavors.

E2 Basics Dressing

RIP ESSELSTYN | *THE ENGINE 2 DIET*

THIS IS ONE of my favorite dressings. My wonderful friend Bridget, who introduced me to the many wonders of vegetarian cooking, whipped it up for me one night in 1996, and my salads have been grateful ever since.

SERVES 2

> **2 tablespoons nutritional yeast**
> **1 tablespoon tamari**
> **1 tablespoon mustard**
> **1 tablespoon balsamic vinegar**
> **Juice of 1 orange, lime, or lemon**
> **1 tablespoon agave nectar, honey, or maple syrup**
> **1 teaspoon vegetarian Worcestershire sauce**
> **1 tablespoon wheat germ**
> **Water to desired consistency**

Whisk the ingredients together in a bowl.

Avocado Dressing

ALAN GOLDHAMER AND DOUG LISLE | *THE HEALTH PROMOTING COOKBOOK*

USE THIS DRESSING when you want a richer touch to your salad. Try replacing the basil with your favorite fresh herb (tarragon, cilantro, oregano, etc.)

MAKES 1 CUP

> ½ **tomato, diced**
> 1 **avocado, peeled and sliced**
> ½ **cup celery juice or water**
> 8 **basil leaves**

Put all ingredients in a blender or food processor and puree until smooth. Serve immediately.

VARIATION:
▶ Replace the basil with your favorite fresh herb (tarragon, cilantro, oregano, etc.).

Yellow Bell Pepper Dressing

MARY MCDOUGALL | THE MCDOUGALL PROGRAM

A BRIGHT-FLAVORED DRESSING with a bit of a kick from the green chiles.

MAKES 3 CUPS

> **Two 12-ounce jars roasted yellow bell peppers**
> 2 **tablespoons diced green chiles**
> 1 **cup water**
> ¼ **cup cider vinegar**
> **Salt and black pepper**

Puree all the ingredients in a blender until smooth.

Hummus–Orange Juice Dressing Plus

ANN CRILE ESSELSTYN | *PREVENT AND REVERSE HEART DISEASE*

THIS IS OUR every-night, quick-to-make salad dressing, which tastes different according to the type of balsamic vinegar and mustard we choose. The hummus helps it feel like a thick dressing. If you don't have nutritional yeast, it will still be good. Using a whole orange is delicious. A good balsamic vinegar makes a difference. Our favorites are Olive Tap vinegars, which come in MANY flavors (tangerine, Sicilian lemon, black currant, traditional, etc.) and are even good by themselves on almost anything.

MAKES ABOUT ½ CUP

> **2 to 3 tablespoons no-tahini hummus**
> **2 tablespoons balsamic vinegar**
> **¼ cup orange juice, or use a whole orange with the sections**
>   **(peel, cut out sections, squeeze juice)**
> **1 tablespoon nutritional yeast**
> **1 teaspoon mustard of your choice**

Mix all the ingredients together.

TIP ▶ For Olive Tap Vinegars, see www.olivetap.com

TIP ▶ You can make your own no-tahini hummus with chickpeas, lemon, and garlic.

Favorite Easy Salad Dressing

BRIAN WENDEL | EXECUTIVE PRODUCER OF *FORKS OVER KNIVES*

TRY THIS IN different combinations to vary the flavor; cashews or walnuts are good options to start with.

Raw nut of your choice (use only one kind)
Orange juice (freshly squeezed is best)
Tomatoes, sliced (optional)

1. Calibrate amounts based on how much dressing you will be serving and the desired creaminess.
2. Blend orange juice, a small amount of the raw nuts, and a few slices of tomato together. Serve over your favorite salad.

TIP ▶ Try using avocado instead of raw nuts for a delicious alternative.

Creamy Golden Gravy

MARY MCDOUGALL | THE MCDOUGALL PROGRAM

THIS GRAVY IS made with brown rice flour instead of wheat flour. The great thing about using rice flour instead of wheat flour for thickening is that it doesn't form lumps like wheat flour often does.

MAKES 2 CUPS

> **2 cups vegetable broth**
> **2 tablespoons low-sodium soy sauce**
> **2 tablespoons tahini**
> **¼ cup brown rice flour**
> **Freshly ground black pepper**

Put the broth, soy sauce, tahini, and flour into a small saucepan. Stir well to mix. Cook over medium-low heat, stirring occasionally, until smooth and thick. Season with black pepper to taste. Serve at once.

TIP ▶ I have walked away and forgotten to stir this gravy, and it still comes out smooth and lump free because of the rice flour.

TIP ▶ This may be made ahead and refrigerated. It will thicken slightly more when refrigerated. To reheat, place in a saucepan, add a small amount of water, whisk to combine, and then heat slowly, stirring occasionally, until hot.

SAUCES AND EASY SNACK IDEAS

Tofu Mayonnaise

MARY MCDOUGALL | THE MCDOUGALL PROGRAM

USE THIS IN place of commercial vegan mayonnaise to greatly reduce the fat without sacrificing the flavor.

MAKES 1½ CUPS

> **One 12.3-ounce package silken tofu**
> **1½ tablespoons lemon juice**
> **1 teaspoon sugar**
> **½ teaspoon salt**
> **½ teaspoon dry mustard**
> **⅛ teaspoon white pepper**

Put all the ingredients into the bowl of a food processor and process until smooth. Store in a covered container in the refrigerator.

Easy Snack Ideas

- Air-popped popcorn—For flavored popcorn, add seasonings or maple syrup
- Brown Rice Snaps with salsa
- Cut veggies with oil-free hummus
- Fresh fruit
- Leftovers
- Homemade trail mix
- Banana with nut butter
- Dried fruit

Fast Pasta and Greens

ANN CRILE ESSELSTYN

USE ANY WHOLE-GRAIN pasta, oil-free pasta sauce, greens, and vegetables you desire. Just be sure to fill that pasta with lots of greens. This is such a good meal in one, and though it takes a number of pots, it is ready very quickly. Skip the zucchini and mushrooms if you are in a hurry.

SERVES 4 TO 6

> One 10-ounce package whole-grain pasta
> One 16-ounce jar pasta sauce (Muir Glen Portobello Mushroom is good and usually available)
> 1 large bunch of kale or collards, roughly chopped, stems removed (6 to 8 cups)
> 1 zucchini, sliced
> 1¾ cups sliced mushrooms

1. Heat a pot of water to boiling. Add the pasta to the water and set a timer for 3 minutes less than the pasta cooking directions recommend. While the pasta is cooking, heat the pasta sauce in a covered saucepan over medium heat until it just begins to bubble. Reduce heat to low and simmer gently until ready to use. When the timer goes off, add the kale to the water and cook about 3 more minutes until the kale is tender.
2. While everything is cooking, put the zucchini in a nonstick skillet over medium heat and dry fry until just brown, then flip the slices over and brown the other side. Push the zucchini to the side, then add the mushrooms and stir-fry until soft. Remove from heat. When pasta and greens are cooked, drain them and put in a large casserole dish. Add the hot pasta sauce and stir. Put mushrooms and zucchini on top and serve.

   TIP ▶ Plenty of pasta sauce is good, so you might need extra pasta sauce.

MAIN DISHES

Raise-the-Roof Sweet Potato–Vegetable Lasagna

RIP ESSELSTYN | *THE ENGINE 2 DIET*

I PREPARED THIS lasagna for my first cooking demonstration at the new Whole Foods Culinary Center in Austin. Tim LaFuente, an award-winning chef who is also an Austin firefighter, asked me to join him at this event, where he made angel hair pasta with chicken, bacon, butter, and oil.

Firefighters are naturally competitive, so the demonstration quickly turned into a contest. No one was declared the winner, but I walked away with my head high because the lasagna was a smashing success: another triumph for plant-happy cuisine!

This lasagna is so good my wife Jill and I chose it to be the main dish at our wedding reception.

SERVES 10 TO 12

> 1 onion, chopped
>
> 1 small head of garlic, all cloves chopped or pressed
>
> 8 ounces mushrooms, sliced
>
> 1 head broccoli, chopped
>
> 2 carrots, chopped
>
> 2 red bell peppers, seeded and chopped
>
> 1 can corn, rinsed and drained
>
> 1 package firm tofu
>
> ½ teaspoon cayenne pepper
>
> 1 teaspoon oregano
>
> 1 teaspoon basil
>
> 1 teaspoon rosemary
>
> 2 jars pasta sauce (kinds with minimal or no added oil)
>
> 2 boxes whole-grain lasagna noodles
>
> 16 ounces frozen spinach, thawed and drained
>
> 2 sweet potatoes, cooked and mashed
>
> 6 Roma tomatoes, sliced thin
>
> 1 cup raw cashews, ground

1. Preheat oven to 400°F. Water sauté the onion and garlic on high heat for 3 minutes in a wok or nonstick pan. Add the mushrooms and cook until the onions are limp and the mushrooms give up their liquid. Remove them to a large bowl with a slotted spoon. Reserve the mushroom liquid in the pan. Water sauté the broccoli and carrots for 5 minutes and add to the mushroom bowl. Sauté the peppers and corn until just beginning

to soften. Add them to the vegetable bowl. Drain the tofu by wrapping in paper towels. Break it up directly in the towel and mix into the vegetable bowl. Add spices to the vegetable bowl and combine.

2. Cover the bottom of a 9 × 13-inch casserole with a layer of sauce. Add a layer of noodles. Cover the noodles with sauce. This way the noodles cook in the oven, saving time and energy. Spread the vegetable mixture over the sauced noodles. Cover with a layer of noodles and another dressing of sauce. Add the spinach to the second layer of sauced noodles. Cover the spinach with the mashed sweet potatoes. Add the final layer of noodles and a last topping of sauce. Cover the lasagna with thinly sliced Roma tomatoes.

3. Cover with foil and bake in the oven for 45 minutes. Remove the foil, sprinkle with the cashews, and return to the oven for 15 minutes. Let sit for 15 minutes before serving.

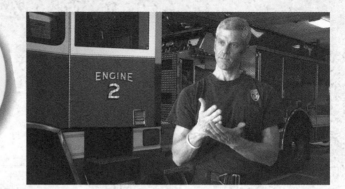

Rip Esselstyn

RIP ESSELSTYN, A former professional firefighter and triathlete, became a standard-bearer for a plant-based diet after an argument lead to a bet. Rip, the eldest son of Dr. Caldwell Esselstyn, worked at the Engine 2 Station in Austin, Texas, for ten years. One day in 2003, he and two other firefighters made a bet about whose cholesterol level was lowest. When they got tested, one of them, James Rae (J.R.), discovered his level was dangerously high. Soon Rip, who had been a plant-based eater since his father published his groundbreaking health study in 1985, decided to help his friend by making Engine 2 a plant-based firehouse. Once J.R. changed his diet along with all the other firefighters, his cholesterol levels plummeted from 344 to a much healthier 196.

Rip then decided to create his own, more formal study to prove the effectiveness of his personal Engine 2 diet, so he recruited fifty-eight people, from firefighters to lawyers, from housewives to doctors, to participate in a six-week program of eating nothing but plant-based meals.

The results were dramatic: Everyone who finished the study lowered his or her cholesterol levels and showed spectacular results on other measures of health as well, from triglyceride levels to weight.

Rip went on to write his best-selling book, *The Engine 2 Diet*, which caught the eye of John Mackey, the CEO of Whole Foods, who in 2010 hired Rip to become a Healthy Eating Partner and to help launch a line of plant-strong foods under the Engine 2 name (the first products—pasta sauces, salad dressings, frozen entrées, and cereals—will be appearing on shelves in mid-2011).

When Rip first switched to a plant-based diet in the 1980s, "it was pretty much considered fringe. Now it's becoming more and more mainstream—in just the last year, a plant-strong diet has seen more television time than ever before: Oprah, Martha Stewart, Ellen DeGeneres, and Dr. Oz have all done shows about it.

"The fact is, as more and more people understand what a plant-based diet is, and why they should do it, it's going to be hard for them to eat the standard American diet of meat, dairy, fat, and more fat. I think we're approaching a point close to where we were with tobacco in the 1950s. Back then, smoking wasn't just accepted, it was encouraged. Even my father, a doctor, felt it was a normal part of life—I remember when my parents had parties, they'd run to the store to buy cigarettes for their guests, and then place ashtrays all over the house.

"I believe that within ten years or so there will be a stigma attached to eating meat similar to the one against smoking today. I wouldn't be surprised if restaurants even start having meat-eating and non-meat-eating sections. And those poor people in the meat-eating sections will look just as pitiful as the people we now see in the smoking sections of public places today, smoking their brains out, looking unhealthy and unhappy."

Layered Tex-Mex Lasagna

MARY MCDOUGALL | THE MCDOUGALL PROGRAM

I HAVE BEEN making and serving variations of this dish for over 20 years. It is one of our family favorites.

SERVES 6 TO 8

TOMATO SAUCE

Two 8-ounce cans tomato sauce

3 cups water

¼ cup cornstarch

3 tablespoons chile powder

½ teaspoon onion powder

¼ teaspoon garlic powder

4 cups mashed cooked pinto beans

1 cup chopped green onions

1½ cups frozen corn kernels, thawed

One 2¼-ounce can sliced black olives, drained, optional

1 to 2 tablespoons chopped green chiles, optional

10 to 12 corn tortillas

Salsa, optional

Tofu sour cream, optional

1. To make the sauce: Put all ingredients for the sauce into a saucepan. Mix well with a whisk until well combined. Cook over medium heat, stirring occasionally, until thickened, about 5 minutes. Taste and add more chile powder if desired. Set aside.
2. To assemble the casserole: Preheat oven to 350°F. Put the beans, green onions, corn, olives and green chiles into a large bowl and mix gently until well combined.
3. Spread 1½ cups of the sauce over the bottom of a oblong nonstick baking dish. Place 3 to 4 corn tortillas in the bottom of the dish. Spread half of the bean mixture evenly over the tortillas. Place another 3 to 4 tortillas over the bean mixture, then spread the remaining bean mixture on top. Cover with 3 to 4 more tortillas, and then pour the remaining sauce over the tortillas. Cover the baking dish with parchment paper, then cover with aluminum foil, crimping the edges over the baking dish. Bake for 45 minutes.

4. Remove the baking dish from oven and let the lasagna rest for about 15 minutes before cutting. Serve with salsa and tofu sour cream, if desired.

TIP ▶ The amount of corn tortillas that you will need depends on the size of your baking dish. Just cover the bottom of the baking dish as well as you can with the first layer of tortillas and then use that same amount for the second and third layers.

E2 Black Beans and Rice

RIP ESSELSTYN | *THE ENGINE 2 DIET*

THIS IS A mainstay dinner dish that is as basic as they come, and oh, so good. Just like my morning bowl of cereal, I've been eating this meal for more than three decades. This is also a great meal to serve when you're having extra guests over for dinner. Serve with healthy chips or warm corn tortillas.

SERVES 3 TO 4

2 cans black beans, rinsed and drained
1 to 1½ cups water or vegetable stock
1 tablespoon Bragg Liquid Aminos
1 teaspoon chile powder
2 to 3 tomatoes, chopped
1 can water chestnuts, drained
1 cup corn, fresh, frozen, or canned
2 red, yellow, or green bell peppers, seeded and chopped
1 bunch cilantro, rinsed and chopped
1 avocado, peeled and sliced
3 cups cooked brown rice
Salsa or tamari to taste

Heat the beans with water or stock, and add the liquid aminos and chile powder. Place the chopped vegetables and cilantro in individual bowls. To serve, place several big spoonfuls of brown rice onto large plates and ladle beans on top. Add generous amounts of chopped vegetables, cilantro, and avocado on top of the beans. Add salsa or tamari to taste.

MexiCali Burritos

JULIEANNA HEVER | THE PLANT-BASED DIETITIAN

THERE'S SOMETHING ABOUT delicious Mexican food in Southern California. These MexiCali Burritos are hearty and decadent and make for a spicy whole-plant food fiesta!

MAKES 4 LARGE OR 8 SMALL BURRITOS

> **One 15-ounce can oil-free refried pinto beans**
> **2 cups frozen corn kernels**
> **1 cup salsa**
> **1 small onion, chopped**
> **½ cup vegetable broth or water**
> **1 teaspoon chili powder**
> **⅓ teaspoon ground cumin**
> **⅓ teaspoon turmeric**
> **⅛ teaspoon cayenne pepper**
> **1 cup nutritional yeast (optional)**
> **4 large or 8 small whole grain tortillas (brown rice, corn, or sprouted wheat)**
> **1 cup shredded lettuce or kale**
> **Guacamole, optional**
> **Tofu-based sour cream, optional**

1. In a large bowl, mash the beans, corn, and salsa with a potato masher.
2. In a large saucepan over medium heat, sauté the onion in the vegetable broth for 5 minutes or until translucent. Add the chili powder, cumin, turmeric, and cayenne and sauté for 1 additional minute.
3. Add the bean mixture and cook, stirring, until heated and smooth, about 5 minutes. Remove from the heat and stir in the nutritional yeast.
4. Meanwhile, heat the tortillas on the stove, flipping every few seconds, until warm. You can also use an oven or toaster oven.
5. Spoon the mixture onto half of one tortilla and top with shredded lettuce. If desired, add guacamole and/or tofu-based sour cream. Fold the tortilla in half, or fold one side over the mixture and then roll to the other side so that the filling is enclosed. Repeat with the remaining tortillas. Serve warm. Store leftovers in an airtight container in the refrigerator.

VARIATION:

► You can turn these into tostadas by leaving the tortillas flat, adding extra lettuce or kale and other salad vegetables (tomatoes, cucumbers, bell peppers), and topping with salsa and/or guacamole.

Wild Rice Stuffed Squash

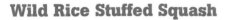

CHEF DEL SROUFE | WELLNESS FORUM FOODS

I GREW UP loving the taste of sage and bread stuffing. It always reminded me of the holidays with family and friends gathered around a big table with lots of really good food. I still love sage stuffing, but now I eat a much healthier version without all of the fat. You can add dried fruit or toasted nuts to this recipe, but I like it as it is prepared below. Try this topped with Creamy Leek Sauce (page 134). You might recognize this dish as the main course in the final scene of *Forks Over Knives*.

SERVES 4

> 2 medium acorn squash, halved and seeded
> 2 medium leeks, trimmed and cut into ½-inch dice
> 2 celery stalks, cut into ½-inch dice
> ½ teaspoon dried sage
> 1 teaspoon poultry seasoning
> ¾ cup wild rice blend
> 1½ cup vegetable broth
> Salt and black pepper to taste

1. Preheat the oven to 350°F.
2. Place the squash halves, cut side down, on a baking sheet. Place the baking sheet in the preheated oven and pour ½ inch of water in the pan. Bake for 25 minutes. Remove from the oven and drain any remaining water from the pan. Turn the squash cut side up and set aside while you prepare the rice.
3. While the squash is baking, heat a 2-quart stockpot over a medium flame. Add the leeks and celery and sauté for 7 to 8 minutes or until the vegetables are tender. Add water 1 to 2 tablespoons at a time to keep the vegetables from sticking. Add the sage, poultry seasoning, rice, and vegetable broth. Cover the pot and bring it to a boil. Reduce to a simmer and cook for 45 minutes, until the rice is tender. Season with salt and pepper.
4. Stuff each squash half with some of the rice. Return the squash to the oven, cover with foil, and bake another 20 minutes.

Creamy Leek Sauce

CHEF DEL SROUFE | WELLNESS FORUM FOODS

THIS SAUCE IS my béchamel sauce. The leeks alone make the sauce, and the pine nuts give it just enough richness to feel indulgent.

SERVES 4

> 2 large leeks, white and light green parts only, thinly sliced and washed
>
> 1 package silken tofu
>
> ½ teaspoon sea salt or to taste
>
> White pepper to taste
>
> 2 tablespoons nutritional yeast
>
> 2 tablespoons toasted pine nuts
>
> Zest of 1 lemon
>
> 4 to 8 tablespoons plain soy milk as needed

1. In a medium saucepan, over a medium flame, sauté the leeks until tender, about 8 minutes. Add water 1 to 2 tablespoons at a time to keep the leeks from sticking. Remove from the flame and add to the bowl of a blender with the remaining ingredients. Puree until smooth and creamy, adding the soy milk as needed to help blend the sauce.
2. Return the sauce to the saucepan and gently heat over a medium flame. Do not boil the sauce.

Rice Stuffed Tomatoes

MATT LEDERMAN AND ALONA PULDE—WITH THANKS TO MONA HOWARD | *KEEP IT SIMPLE, KEEP IT WHOLE*

TOTALLY WORTH A little extra work! No one can resist these tomatoes. You will be sorry you don't have more left over.

SERVES 6

6 large very ripe tomatoes, at room temperature

1½ cups sliced mushrooms

1 cup chopped onion

Vegetable broth

One 10-ounce package of frozen chopped spinach, thawed and drained

2 medium avocados, mashed

2 teaspoons minced garlic

1 teaspoon basil

1 teaspoon brown sugar or agave nectar

½ teaspoon salt

¼ teaspoon black pepper

½ cup quick-cooking rice

¼ cup plus 2 tablespoons Parma! (vegan "Parmesan cheese"), optional

1. Preheat oven to 400°F.
2. Cut a slice from the top of each tomato and scoop out the pulp, leaving a ¼-inch-thick shell; set aside. Chop the tomato pulp (makes about 3½ cups) and set aside.
3. Sauté the mushrooms and onion in some vegetable broth in a large skillet over high heat. Cook, stirring, until tender, about 10 minutes. Add spinach, avocados, reserved chopped tomatoes, garlic, basil, sugar, salt, and pepper. Cook over low heat, stirring occasionally, until flavors blend, about 10 minutes. Stir in the rice, remove from heat, cover, and let stand for 5 minutes. Stir in ¼ cup of the Parma!
4. Place the tomato shells in a 13 × 9 × 2-inch baking pan. Spoon the hot mixture into the shells, dividing evenly. Sprinkle 1 teaspoon Parma! on top of each. Bake until the tomatoes are hot and the filling is golden, about 15 minutes.

TIP ▶ Parma! Vegan Parmesan is a natural seasoning with only whole-food ingredients and no oils: www.eatintheraw.com/ingredients.php. If you can't get Parma!, a sprinkling of nutritional yeast is the perfect "cheesy" alternative.

VARIATION:
▶ Replace the frozen, thawed spinach with about 1 cup chopped cooked spinach.

Steamed Veggies and Tofu with Brown Rice

RORY FREEDMAN AND KIM BARNOUIN | *SKINNY BITCH IN THE KITCH*

THIS DISH TASTES so simple, pure, and good it's one of my staples. I like to make a big pot of rice and big batch of tahini ahead of time. Then, when I'm in a hurry for a fast, healthy meal, all I need to do is toss some veggies in the steamer and I'm good to go.—*Rory Freedman*

SERVES 4 TO 6

> 1½ cups medium-grain brown rice
>
> 3½ cups water, plus more for steaming
>
> ¼ teaspoon fine sea salt
>
> ½ cup tahini (sesame seed paste)
>
> ¼ cup plus 2 tablespoons Bragg Liquid Aminos, plus more for the table
> (or 4 tablespoons tamari or soy sauce)
>
> 2 carrots, cut into ¼-inch slices
>
> ¼ head cauliflower, cut into bite-sized florets (about 2 cups)
>
> ¼ head red cabbage (about 6 ounces), cut into ¼-inch strips
>
> ¼ bunch kale (about 4 ounces or four to six leaves), cut into ½-inch strips
>
> 1 broccoli crown, cut into bite-size florets (about 2½ cups)
>
> 7 to 8 ounces firm or extra firm tofu cut into ¼-inch slices, then cut on a diagonal into triangles
>
> ¼ cup raw pine nuts

1. In a 2-quart saucepan over high heat, combine the rice, 3 cups of the water, and the salt. Bring to a boil, reduce the heat to a simmer, cover, and cook until the water is absorbed and the rice is tender, about 45 minutes. Remove from the heat and let the rice stand, covered, at least 10 minutes.

2. Meanwhile, in a small bowl, whisk together the tahini, ¼ cup of the Bragg Liquid Aminos (or 8 teaspoons of tamari or soy sauce), and the remaining ½ cup of water; set aside. If the dressing is too thick, slowly stir in more water as needed.

3. In a pot fitted with a steamer insert, bring 1 inch of water and the remaining 2 tablespoons of Bragg Liquid Aminos (or 4 teaspoons of the tamari or soy sauce) to a boil. Arrange the carrots and cauliflower in the insert and steam for 3 minutes. Add the cabbage, kale, broccoli, and tofu and steam for 3 minutes, until the vegetables are tender and the tofu is heated through. To serve, place the rice on plates or a platter and top with the vegetable mixture, tahini sauce, and pine nuts. Pass any remaining sauce and additional Bragg Liquid Aminos at the table.

Plant-Powered Polenta Pizza

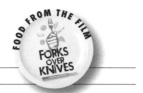

MOIRA NORDHOLT | THE FEEL GOOD GURU

THIS EASY AND fun wheat-free pie also makes a wonderful appetizer or finger food, cut into small wedges and served warm from the oven.

Don't be intimidated thinking you'll have to stand over the stove stirring constantly for an hour to make your polenta crust. With this easy-shmeasy version, you whip it up, cover it, and walk away. The polenta takes the shape and size of the pan you cook it in and then browns in the oven on a cookie sheet. Simply top with your favorite sauce and toppings, or follow the recipe below for a perfect vegan polenta pizza!

The tomato sauce can be made in advance.

MAKES 4 LARGE SLICES

HEIRLOOM TOMATO SAUCE

1 pound heirloom tomatoes

Sea salt

6 to 8 garlic cloves

Fresh herbs, such as basil, chives, oregano, and sage

POLENTA CRUST

4 cups water or unsalted vegetable broth

1 teaspoon sea salt

2 cups organic polenta or cornmeal

HERBED CASHEW "CHEESE," OPTIONAL

1 cup organic cashews

½ lemon, juiced

1 teaspoon Himalayan sea salt

1 teaspoon fresh basil or your favorite seasonal herb

¼ cup spring water

Seasonal toppings of your choice, such as finely sliced red onions, zucchini rounds, sun-dried tomatoes, thinly sliced Chinese eggplant, or fresh baby artichokes

Fresh basil

1. For the tomato sauce: Preheat the oven to 350°F. Quarter the heirloom tomatoes and place faceup on a roasting pan. Sprinkle with sea salt. Add the whole cloves of garlic and roast for 30 minutes or until lightly caramelized. Scrape the roasted tomatoes and garlic into a bowl and

pulse with an immersion blender or mash with a fork. Chop some of your favorite seasonal fresh herbs and stir in.

2. For the crust: Bring the water and sea salt to a boil in a 10- or 12-inch pot or sauté pan. Whisk in the polenta slowly until all is incorporated. Stir for about 1 minute, then turn the heat to low, cover the pot, and leave it for 40 minutes. Turn off the heat and allow to sit for another 10 minutes.

3. Preheat the oven to 350°F.

4. Carefully turn the pot upside down, dropping the polenta onto a cutting board. Slice the polenta in half, parallel to the cutting board, into two round pizza crusts. Place the crusts onto a cookie sheet and bake for about 30 minutes, or until crispy around the edges.

5. For the cashew "cheese": Put all the "cheese" ingredients into a food processor and puree, adding water slowly, until they reach a thick, cream-cheese-like consistency. (You want to be able to form little "cheese balls," so be careful not to add too much water.) Adjust seasonings to taste. (I enjoy a clove or two of garlic and sometimes more lemon juice, depending how juicy the lemon is.)

6. Assemble the pizza: Spread the tomato sauce over the polenta crust, then use a teaspoon to form little balls of the cashew "cheese" and arrange them on top. Add toppings of choice.

7. Bake the pizza for 10 minutes just to heat the toppings. Garnish with whole fresh basil leaves and serve.

VARIATIONS:

▶ To use almonds instead of cashews, first soak them overnight in spring water.

▶ Try maple shiitakes as a topping: Toss sliced shiitake mushrooms in a cast iron frying pan with a splash of tamari and a splash of maple syrup. Cook over medium heat until the liquid is absorbed.

Creamy Noodle Casserole

ELISE MURPHY | T. COLIN CAMPBELL FOUNDATION

THIS CASSEROLE SATISFIES cravings for comfort food, and is a pleaser for plant-based eaters and non-plant-based eaters alike. It's also good reheated.

SERVES 10

16 ounces whole-wheat pasta: farfalle, penne, or other short pasta

1 large yellow onion, chopped

2 large carrots, chopped

2 celery stalks, chopped

8 ounces green beans, cut into pieces

16 ounces cooked cannellini beans

1 cup shelled peas

5 cups vegetable broth, separated

½ cup whole-wheat flour

⅓ cup minced fresh parsley

2 teaspoons dried thyme

2 teaspoons paprika

1 cup nondairy Portobello mushroom broth, or additional vegetable broth

Salt and pepper, to taste

1 cup panko bread crumbs

1. Preheat the oven to 350°F. Cook the pasta in a pot of boiling water until just underdone. Drain, return to the pot, and set aside.
2. In a large skillet over medium heat, sauté the onion, carrots, and celery in water. Cook, stirring occasionally, until softened, about 5 minutes. Stir in the green beans, cannellini beans, and peas. Cook for another 4 to 5 minutes.
3. Combine the vegetables and pasta and spread in a deep 9 × 13-inch casserole dish.
4. In a medium saucepan over medium heat, add ½ cup of the vegetable broth and quickly whisk in the flour. Slowly whisk in the remaining broth. Add the parsley, thyme, paprika, and mushroom broth. Season with salt and pepper to taste. Cook, stirring until thickened.
5. Pour the sauce over the noodle-vegetable mixture, and bake, covered, for 30 minutes.
6. Remove the casserole from the oven, uncover, and sprinkle panko evenly on top. Return to the oven and bake, uncovered, for 10 minutes, until the panko is nicely browned. Serve hot.

Kathmandu Stew

MOIRA NORDHOLT | THE FEEL GOOD GURU

THIS IS A nice, mildly curried, mildly sweet red lentil and yam stew that's satisfying served alone or with a simple raita made with soy yogurt, toasted cumin seeds, and cucumbers.

SERVES 4

- **1 teaspoon cumin seeds**
- **1 teaspoon cumin powder**
- **1 teaspoon fennel seeds**
- **3 teaspoon curry powder**
- **½ teaspoon coriander powder**
- **½ teaspoon turmeric powder**
- **1 pinch of cinnamon**
- **2 cups organic red lentils, rinsed**
- **1 medium sweet potato, diced**
- **2 carrots, diced**
- **1 medium red onion, diced**
- **4 garlic cloves, minced**
- **1 or 2 teaspoons sambal oelek (chile paste) or dried red chiles**
- **4 cups water**
- **Pink Himalayan sea salt**
- **1 small bunch of fresh cilantro, chopped**

1. Toast the cumin seeds and powder, fennel seeds, curry powder, coriander, turmeric, and cinnamon in a cast iron frying pan on high heat until the cumin seeds start to pop.
2. Add the red lentils and stir until the spices are mixed in. Add a splash of water and continue cooking and stirring. Add the sweet potato, carrots, onion, sambal oelek, and 4 cups water.
3. Stir, cover, and bring to a boil, then stir again, turn down the heat, and simmer for about 20 minutes until the sweet potatoes and lentils are cooked. Add salt to taste, and serve garnished with fresh cilantro.

Mushrooms, Kale, and Potatoes

MARY MCDOUGALL | THE MCDOUGALL PROGRAM

KALE IS A very nutritious vegetable, loaded with phytonutrients. This is delicious, healthy, and quick to put together and makes a complete meal for John and myself. We like this with Sriracha Hot Chili Sauce over the top for even more heat.

SERVES 2 TO 3

> **3 cups chunked Yukon Gold or red potatoes**
> **2 onions, chopped**
> **2 garlic cloves, minced**
> **4 to 5 cups chopped exotic mushrooms (see tip)**
> **6 cups packed, coarsely chopped dinosaur kale, stems removed**
> **2 tablespoons soy sauce**
> **1 to 2 teaspoons chile paste**
> **Freshly ground black pepper**

1. Put the potatoes in a saucepan with enough water to cover. Bring to a boil, reduce heat, and cook until fairly tender, about 8 minutes. Drain and set aside.
2. Meanwhile, put the onion, garlic, and mushrooms in a large nonstick sauté pan or wok. Do not add any liquid. Dry-fry over medium heat, stirring frequently, for about 5 to 6 minutes, until onions and mushrooms are fairly tender. Add the kale and stir gently to combine. Continue to cook, stirring frequently for about 2 minutes. Add the cooked potatoes. Cook, stirring occasionally, for about 3 more minutes, then add the soy sauce, chile paste, and pepper to taste. Cook for 3 to 5 minutes, until kale is tender and potatoes are somewhat browned. Serve warm.

TIP ▶ Use any assortment of firm small potatoes or fingerlings, cut into bite-size pieces. Watch them carefully during boiling: don't let them get overcooked.

TIP ▶ Assorted exotic mushrooms, such as clamshell, trumpet, oyster, and chanterelle, are available in most markets. Uses about 1 pound.

TIP ▶ If you can't get dinosaur kale (also called Lacinato Blue), use regular kale. To easily remove the stems from any kind of kale, grasp the bottom of the stem with one hand, gently but firmly grasp the leafy part with your other hand, and pull upward along the stem.

Polenta with Rice and Beans

KAREN CAMPBELL | THE CAMPBELL FAMILY

THIS DISH GOES well with a tossed salad, broccoli, or cooked greens. Enjoy!

SERVES 4

POLENTA CRUST

2 cups boiling water

¾ cup polenta

¼ teaspoon salt

1 cup low-sodium, no-fat vegetable broth (I like the one by Pacific Natural Foods)

1 cup water

One 14½-ounce can diced tomatoes

1 small diced onion

1 cup short-grain brown rice

1 tablespoon chile powder

One 15½-ounce can black beans, drained and rinsed

½ cup fat-free, low-sodium salsa

1 avocado, mashed

4 teaspoons lemon juice

½ teaspoon garlic powder

1. For the polenta crust: Bring the water to a boil and whisk in the polenta and salt. Cook, stirring constantly, for 10 to 12 minutes until the polenta pulls away from the side of the pan. Dump the cooked polenta into a large pie dish and spread evenly over the bottom and sides of the dish. Set aside.

2. Combine the broth, water, tomatoes, onion, rice, and chile powder in a rice cooker or saucepan. Cook until all liquid is gone and rice is tender, about 45 minutes. Preheat oven to 350°F.

3. After the rice is cooked, stir in the black beans. Spread the rice-bean mixture evenly in the polenta crust. Spread salsa over the rice-bean mixture. Bake for 30 minutes. Remove from the oven and set aside for 5 to 10 minutes.

4. Meanwhile, mash the avocado in a small bowl with the lemon juice and garlic powder. Slice the pie, and put a dollop of avocado mixture (about 1 tablespoon) on each slice before serving.

TIP ▶ Short-grain rice sticks together better than long- and medium-grain rice.

Mini Polenta Pies with Spinach Walnut Stuffing Served with Spicy Tomato Sauce

DARSHANA THACKER | AYURVEDIC VEGAN CHEF

THIS DISH BLENDS different colors, textures, and aromas into a culinary burst of flavors with every bite. You can also make it as a casserole.

SERVES 4

THE POLENTA

- **1 cup polenta**
- **½ teaspoon cumin seeds**
- **6 cups water**
- **1 teaspoon salt**

THE STUFFING

- **½ cup water**
- **½ cup finely chopped onions**
- **1 teaspoon grated fresh ginger**
- **1 teaspoon minced garlic**
- **1 teaspoon green chiles**
- **1 teaspoon ground cumin**
- **½ teaspoon salt**
- **1 cup chopped kale**
- **4 cup finely chopped fresh spinach**
- **½ cup coarsely ground walnuts**

THE TOMATO SAUCE

- **2 cups diced tomatoes**
- **¼ cup grated red onions**
- **½ teaspoon minced garlic**
- **½ teaspoon Italian herb mix**
- **1 teaspoon salt**
- **½ teaspoon turmeric**
- **½ teaspoon chile powder**
- **1 tablespoon finely chopped fresh basil**

1. For the polenta: Heat the water in a pot or kettle. Roast the cumin seeds lightly in a sauté pan, add the polenta, and roast for 2 more minutes. Pour the hot water gently over the polenta and stir. Cook on low heat

for 7 to 10 minutes, stirring occasionally, until the polenta is completely cooked and all the water has been absorbed.

2. Spread the polenta evenly on a flat dish to about ¾ inch thick. Let it cool completely. With a large round cookie cutter, cut out patties. You should get 8 patties. Set aside.

3. For the stuffing: Put the water and onions in a sauté pan and cook until soft, 5 to 10 minutes. Let the water cook off completely. Add the ginger, garlic, green chiles, cumin, and salt and cook for another 2 minutes. Add the kale and spinach and cook until the spinach has wilted. Add the walnuts, mix well, and cook for another 1 to 2 minutes. Set aside.

4. For the tomato sauce: Boil the tomatoes in a pot of water until the skin softens and splits. Drain and cut into fine pieces. Put the onions and garlic into a sauté pan and cook with a small amount of water until translucent. Add the Italian herbs, salt, turmeric, and chile powder and stir. Add the tomatoes. Cook for 10 minutes and remove from heat. Puree the sauce in a blender until smooth.

5. Return the sauce to the sauté pan and reheat. Just before serving, add the chopped basil.

6. To assemble the pie: Preheat the oven to 350°F. Place four of the polenta patties in a baking dish. Top with the stuffing, divided evenly among the patties. Place the remaining polenta patties on top, and bake the pies for 20 to 25 minutes. Top with hot tomato sauce and serve.

Caribbean Rundown

CHRISTY MORGAN | THE BLISSFUL CHEF

THIS DISH IS sort of like gumbo. In the Caribbean they call it "rundown" because they throw whatever they can find into this tasty stew seasoned with jerk spices. This is wonderful served with coconut rice, black beans, and plantains.

SERVES 4 TO 5

½ cup water
1 tablespoon chopped fresh thyme
1 teaspoon chopped fresh oregano
1 cup carrot, chopped
2 cups chopped asparagus
2 cups chopped chayote squash
1 tablespoon jerk seasonings
Salt
1 cup chopped collards
½ cup frozen peas
½ cup veggie broth
Small can tomato sauce
Soy sauce or tamari

Bring the water to a boil in a medium skillet. Stir in the thyme, oregano, carrot, asparagus, chayote, jerk seasonings, and a pinch of salt. Cover and simmer for 5 minutes, stirring occasionally. Add the collards, peas, and veggie broth and stir well. Cover and cook for 10 minutes, stirring occasionally. Add the tomato sauce, cover, and simmer for another 5 minutes. Add soy sauce or tamari to taste and simmer for another few minutes.

Minty-Lemon Lentils with Spinach

ANN CRILE ESSELSTYN

THE MINT MAKES this absolutely delicious and is worth a special trip to the store to find. Better yet GROW your own. Use as much spinach as possible. It melts to nothing. Swiss chard also works well and cooks almost as quickly as spinach. Red lentils cook fast. If you use other lentils, you will need to cook them longer. Lime juice adds an especially good flavor. Sweet potatoes are BEAUTIFUL in here! This is so good, I usually double the recipe, and even that is not enough!

This can be served with broccoli or fresh asparagus and sliced tomatoes.

SERVES 2 TO 4

2 garlic cloves, chopped

3 cups low-sodium vegetable broth

1 cup red lentils

3 medium red-skinned potatoes or 1 large sweet potato, cut into ½-inch dice (2 to 3 cups)

6 to 12 ounces baby spinach leaves (you can't have too much)

Zest of 1 lemon or lime

3 tablespoons lemon or lime juice

⅛ to ¼ teaspoon cayenne

¼ cup fresh mint, chopped

Black pepper

Cook garlic for 1 minute in a saucepan over medium heat, adding a little vegetable broth or water as necessary. Add the 3 cups vegetable broth, lentils, and potatoes and bring to a boil. Reduce heat, cover, and simmer for 10 to 15 minutes until the lentils are tender. Add spinach, lemon zest, lemon juice, and cayenne. Cover and simmer until spinach wilts, about 2 minutes. Stir in mint and add black pepper to taste.

Seared Red Lentil Pâté

ANASTASIA ST. JOHN | COMPASSIONATE DIET AND LIFESTYLE ADVOCATE

THIS IS A fun and delicious way to prepare lentils. It's a great entrée for a special dinner.

SERVES 4

> 1 cup red lentils
> 3 cups water
> ½ cup chopped onion
> 1 cup chopped cremini mushrooms
> ½ cup raw cashews
> 1 garlic clove, minced
> ½ teaspoon sea salt
> ¼ teaspoon black pepper
> ⅛ teaspoon cayenne
> ½ teaspoon thyme
> 1 teaspoon rosemary

1. Bring the red lentils and water to a boil in a medium pot. Reduce the heat and simmer until the lentils are soft, about 15 minutes. Drain off extra water if necessary.
2. Cook the onion and mushrooms in a cast iron skillet until browned. Put the cooked lentils, onion, and mushrooms into a blender. Add the cashews, garlic, salt, pepper, cayenne, thyme, and rosemary and puree until smooth. Spread the pâté evenly over the bottom of an 8 × 8-inch glass baking pan and allow to cool, then refrigerate at least 2 hours or until firm.
3. Cut the pâté into four squares, then brown each side in the cast iron skillet over medium-high heat. Serve immediately.

Lentil Loaf

CHEF AJ | *UNPROCESSED*

YOU WON'T FIND soy or breadcrumbs in this loaf, just whole-food goodness.

SERVES 8

> 3 cups cooked lentils (about 1 pound after cooking)
> One 16-ounce bag of frozen carrots, defrosted and drained (about 3 cups)
> 2 cups chopped red onion (about 1 large)
> 2 garlic cloves, peeled
> ½ cup fresh Italian parsley
> 2 cups raw walnuts
> 2 cups uncooked oats (not instant)
> 2 tablespoons sun-dried tomato powder
> 1 teaspoon poultry seasoning, optional

1. Preheat oven to 350°F.
2. Put the lentils, carrots, onion, garlic, parsley, 1 cup of the walnuts, and 1 cup of the oats in a food processor fitted with the "S" blade. Pulse until combined, then continue to process until almost pastelike. (Depending on the size of your food processor you may have to do this in several batches.) Scrape the mixture into a bowl.
3. Chop the remaining 1 cup walnuts and add it to the lentil mixture along with the remaining 1 cup oats, the tomato powder, and the poultry seasoning. Stir to mix well.
4. Scrape the mixture into a silicone standard loaf pan and bake, uncovered, for 50 to 55 minutes until golden brown. Remove from the oven and let sit at least 10 minutes, then invert onto a serving dish. Decorate with whole walnuts, if desired. Let cool another 5 minutes and then slice.

TIP▶ If you do not have a food processor, you can chop all the ingredients finely by hand and use a potato masher to incorporate the lentils. Your loaf will have a chunkier texture.

VARIATIONS:

▶ This loaf is delicious even without any sauce or gravy of any kind, but you can also add your favorite condiments, such as ketchup, mustard, or barbecue sauce.

▶ Stuff cold leftovers into pita pockets for a great lunch!

Garbanzo Bean Loaf

ALAN GOLDHAMER AND DOUG LISLE | *THE HEALTH PROMOTING COOKBOOK*

A GREAT CHOICE when you want a filling, substantial main dish. The leftovers can be used for sandwiches.

SERVES 8

>4 cups cooked, blended garbanzo beans
>2 cups cooked brown rice
>2 cups tomato sauce
>1 tablespoon dry mustard
>1 cup grated carrots
>Juice of ½ lemon

1. Preheat oven to 350°F. In a large mixing bowl, combine the blended beans and rice. Add the tomato sauce, mustard, carrots, and lemon juice.
2. Spoon into a loaf pan, and bake for 30 minutes. Cover the loaf with aluminum foil if the top begins to brown too quickly.

VARIATION:

▶ Add 1½ teaspoons garlic powder or onion powder with the other seasonings.

Lima Bean Surprise

MARY MCDOUGALL | THE MCDOUGALL PROGRAM

THIS IS ONE of my favorite fast and delicious meals that can be put together, cooked, and served in only 15 minutes.

SERVES 3 TO 4

¼ cup vegetable broth

½ tablespoon soy sauce

2½ cups frozen lima beans (16-ounce bag)

2½ cups shredded cabbage

1 to 2 teaspoons seasoning mixture (see tip)

½ to 1 teaspoon sambal oelek (chile paste)

1½ cups frozen corn, thawed slightly

2½ to 3 cups cooked brown rice

1 large chopped tomato

Put broth, soy sauce, lima beans, and shredded cabbage in a large nonstick sauté pan and cook, stirring frequently, for about 2 minutes. Add the seasoning mixture of your choice and the sambal oelek. [...]e to cook for another 3 minutes. Add corn and cook, stirring [...]ally, for 2 minutes. Add the rice and continue to cook and stir [...] rice is heated through and all the vegetables are tender. Stir in [...]s. Serve at once.

[...]gs of shredded cabbage are available in many supermarkets, or you [...] your own cabbage in a food processor. To thaw the corn slightly, [...] colander and rinse with cool water.

TIP ▶ If you don't have leftover cooked rice in your refrigerator, you can heat a package of frozen brown rice in the microwave.

TIP ▶ There are many delicious seasoning mixtures on the market. Try Mrs. Dash or a lemon-dill mixture. I often use Lemony Dill Zest Seasoning by Vegetarian Express. We like to top this with Sriracha Hot Chili Sauce, and it is wonderful rolled up in a soft corn tortilla.

Quick Barbequed Tempeh

JO STEPANIAK | *BREAKING THE FOOD SEDUCTION* BY NEAL BARNARD, MD

THIS INCREDIBLY SIMPLE dish is a fabulous choice for the outdoor grill. In cool weather cook it on an indoor grill or in the oven. Leftovers make a great sandwich filling.

SERVES 4

> **16 ounces tempeh**
> **1 large onion, halved and thinly sliced**
> **2 cups bottled barbecue sauce**

Cut tempeh into 1-inch chunks. Steam over boiling water for 15 minutes. Place tempeh and sliced onion in a deep glass or ceramic dish and pour barbecue sauce over all. Toss gently and marinate in refrigerator for at least 1 hour. Cook on outdoor or indoor grill until browned and heated through. Baste frequently with barbecue sauce. Alternatively, bake in a covered casserole dish in a 350°F oven for 30 minutes.

Kale-Lemon Sandwiches, the Ultimate in Health

ANN CRILE ESSELSTYN

WE HAD BEEN traveling and longed for GREENS, and when we got home only KALE was in the refrigerator. Lucky us for that day! This sandwich is stunningly delicious and tastes as good as it is healthy. Any greens you choose will work. The lemon adds an almost sweet taste. Be generous with it!

SERVES 2 TO 4

> 4 slices of dense, whole-grain bread
> ½ to 1 lemon
> 1 bunch of kale, chopped into bite-size pieces, stems removed (4 cups or more)
> No-tahini hummus (see tip)
> 4 green onions, chopped
> ½ bunch of fresh cilantro or parsley, chopped
> 1 large tomato, sliced into 4 thick slices, optional

1. Toast bread well. If using a very dense bread or a rye or pumpernickel double or even triple toast. Make it almost cracker-like. Cut the ends off the lemon, zest them, then squeeze the juice from the ends into a bowl with the zest. Discard the ends. VERY thinly slice the main part of the lemon and set aside.
2. Put kale in a pot with 3 to 4 inches of water in the bottom. Bring to a boil, cover, and cook until tender, 3 to 5 minutes; check frequently. Kale is good when cooked to an almost spinachlike tenderness. Drain well, shaking the strainer until all water is gone, then sprinkle the kale in the strainer with the reserved lemon zest and juice. LOTS of lemon makes this good!
3. Spread the toast thickly with hummus, sprinkle with green onions, pile cilantro on top of the green onions, and then place lemon slices over the cilantro. Put a big handful of lemony kale on top. It is delicious just like that, or top with a tomato slice. And there you have it: health in a bite! A bit of a messy one at that!

TIP▶ Hummus is easy to make yourself by pureeing a base of chickpeas, lemon, and garlic and then adding cumin, vinegar, red peppers, parsley, or cilantro to taste.

VARIATION:
▶ Substitute Swiss chard or greens of your choice for the kale.

Raise the Flag Lunch

ANTHONY YEN | FEATURED IN *FORKS OVER KNIVES*

THIS IS ONE of my most frequently used meals. I never get tired of it.

SERVES 1

1 portobello mushroom

Cooked brown or wild rice

Salsa

1 fresh tomato, chopped

Prepared horseradish

Clean the portobello well and remove the stem. Mix some cooked rice with salsa and fresh chopped tomato at whatever proportions you prefer. Scoop the mixture into the portobello cap and place it in a rice cooker or a steamer basket over a pot of boiling water. Steam until the portobello is soft. Add a little horseradish on top for extra kick.

VARIATION:

▶ Alternatively, you can bake the stuffed portobello. Preheat the oven to 350°F and cook on a baking sheet until soft.

Incredible Tomatoes and Cucumbers

MICAELA COOK | T. COLIN CAMPBELL FOUNDATION

EATING TOMATOES AND cucumbers with this no-oil version of a vinaigrette is so simple and tasty. It's also a great way to use up garden produce in the summer, instead of handing your neighbors bags of tomatoes!

SERVES 5

3 large tomatoes

2 medium cucumbers

3 tablespoons apple cider vinegar

3 tablespoons agave or rice syrup

3 tablespoons mustard

Salt to taste

Wash the tomatoes and cucumbers. If you don't mind the flavor of the cucumber skin, don't worry about peeling them. Chop the tomatoes and cucumbers into medium-small cubes. Add the vinegar, syrup, and mustard and toss. Taste before salting in case you don't want salt, but if you do, salt to taste and toss again. Serve chilled. If this can marinate in the refrigerator beforehand the flavors will be more delicious.

Stewed Tomatoes

KAREN CAMPBELL | THE CAMPBELL FAMILY

THIS IS DELICIOUS over potatoes, biscuits, or cornbread.

SERVES 4

¼ cup diced onions

¼ cup dried green bell peppers

¼ teaspoon sea salt

1 teaspoon Italian seasoning

½ teaspoon garlic powder

¼ cup water

One 14½-ounce can diced tomatoes or 4 medium-to-large tomatoes,
   diced or blended

1½ teaspoons sweetener

3 tablespoons whole wheat flour

½ cup soy milk

Black pepper

1. Add the onions, bell peppers, salt, Italian seasoning, garlic, and water to a sauté pan and cook for 5 minutes. Add the tomatoes and sweetener and bring to a boil.
2. Whisk the flour with the milk in a small bowl until smooth. Add flour and milk to the hot tomato mixture and cook, stirring, until thick. Add black pepper to taste.

Green Beans with Tarragon

KAREN CAMPBELL | THE CAMPBELL FAMILY

I LOVE THIS quick method to dress up green beans.

SERVES 4

> **1½ pound green beans**
> **1½ cups water**
> **One 6-ounce package mushrooms, sliced**
> **2 to 3 garlic cloves, minced**
> **1 teaspoon tarragon**
> **½ teaspoon sea salt**

Wash the beans and snap them in half. Put beans, water, mushrooms, garlic, tarragon, and salt into a skillet and cook until the beans are tender.

Eggplant Dengaku

ISA CHANDRA MOSKOWITZ | *APPETITE FOR REDUCTION*

A STAPLE ON Japanese restaurant menus, this eggplant is broiled and coated in a rich, pungent, and slightly sweet miso sauce. I'm not usually a stickler for a particular type of miso, but here I insist that you use red miso for the most authentic taste. And by authentic I mean Japanese-American restaurant authentic, because I'm just a nice Jewish girl who has never actually been to Japan. Serve this over brown rice.

SERVES 4

> ¼ cup mirin
> 2 teaspoons soy sauce
> 2 tablespoons water
> 5 teaspoons agave
> ¼ cup red miso
> 2 pounds eggplant, cut ½-inch thick
> Sliced scallions, for garnish (optional)

1. In a saucepot, combine the mirin, soy sauce, and agave. Bring to a boil and then lower the heat. Add the agave and miso. Stir over very low heat, whisking often, until it is smooth.
2. Preheat the broiler and place a rack about 6 inches from the heat. Spray a large-rimmed baking sheet with nonstick cooking spray. Arrange the eggplant slices in a single layer and spray lightly with cooking spray. Broil for about 6 minutes; the tops should be browned and the eggplant should be cooked but still a bit firm. Remove from the oven.
3. Use a tablespoon to divide the miso sauce among all the eggplant slices, then use the back of the spoon to spread it on each entire slice. Place back in the broiler and broil for 2 more minutes. The miso should be a little bubbly. Serve as soon as you can.

Asparagus Red Pepper Stir-Fry

CHEF DEL SROUFE | WELLNESS FORUM FOODS

STIR-FRYING IS AN Asian technique for cooking meat and vegetables quickly so that they retain their texture and flavor. In this recipe you can be creative and substitute other vegetables, such as snow peas and fresh, thinly sliced carrots, for the asparagus.

SERVES 3 TO 4

1 pound fresh asparagus, trimmed and cut into 1-inch pieces

1 red bell pepper, cut into ¼-inch-thick slivers

8 ounces cremini mushrooms, thinly sliced

2 garlic cloves, minced

1 tablespoon Bragg Liquid Aminos

Heat a large skillet over high heat and add the asparagus, bell pepper, and mushrooms. Stir-fry for 4 to 5 minutes, adding water 1 to 2 tablespoons at a time to keep the vegetables from sticking. Add the garlic and cook another minute. Add the Liquid Aminos and toss well. Serve immediately.

Kale Greens

YOANNAH BROWN | SOUL VEGETARIAN EAST RESTAURANT, CHICAGO

AN EASY WAY to make greens taste delicious, this dish is a favorite of Dr. Terry Mason. The flavor is savory and goes with any meal theme.

SERVES 4

¼ cup water

12 cups kale, washed and coarsely chopped

1 cup chopped onion

1 tablespoon garlic powder

¼ cup nutritional yeast

¼ cup of Bragg Liquid Aminos

Heat the water in a large pot until it comes to a boil. Add the kale, onion, garlic powder, and nutritional yeast. Cover and let cook until the kale is soft and tender, about 15 minutes. Add Liquid Aminos to taste and mix thoroughly.

Kale with Miraculous Walnut Sauce

ANN CRILE ESSELSTYN | *PREVENT AND REVERSE HEART DISEASE*

WHEN WE VISIT our son, Rip, in Austin, Texas, we always eat at Casa de Luz, a macrobiotic restaurant, because we love the food and especially the walnut sauce on kale. In the past, kale had been one of our last-choice greens. We asked the cook for the walnut sauce recipe they put on kale and we learned two things: First, boil kale in lots of water (and now we love kale even without the sauce). And second, the three ingredients for the sauce: walnuts, garlic, and tamari. The result, something shockingly delicious and totally different from the individual ingredients! People need to learn to make kale and put walnut sauce on it. This sauce is NOT for those with heart disease unless used VERY sparingly. Although it is best to make this according to your own taste, here is a possible recipe:

1 bunch kale, prepared (see next page)
1 to 2 tablespoons low-sodium tamari
½ cup water, or more depending on preference for thick or thin
½ cup walnuts
1 garlic clove

1. Put in a blender or food processor a handful of walnuts, a clove or more of garlic depending on garlic tolerance, and a big sprinkle of low-sodium tamari.
2. Blend and add as much water as necessary (about ½ cup) to make it the right consistency to pour over the kale. It can be quite thin to be good and it goes a long way. It is good on absolutely everything.

How to Prepare Kale

1. Remove the stems from the kale, keeping the leaves whole. The most fun way to do this is as follows (this works well for collards too):

   - Hold the spine of the kale firmly in your right hand.
   - Loosely hold the lower part of the spine, just below the leafy greens, in your left hand. You may need to tear back the lower leaves to expose some of the stem.
   - Holding firmly with your right hand and lightly with your left, move your hands apart. The greens will end up in your left hand and the bare stem in your right. (Collard spines do not always come away as far up the leaf, but that doesn't matter.)

2. Now chop the pile of greens into bite-size pieces. (Don't waste the spines; assemble them all in a row, chop them into tiny pieces, optionally boil them, and add them to soup!)
3. Boil about 1½ inches of water in a large frying pan and spread out the kale greens in the pan. Cover and cook for 5 minutes, then test to see if it is cooked to your liking. Like spinach, kale is best if it is a little more cooked—but don't overcook it.
4. Remove from the heat, drain, and serve, or proceed to use the kale in another recipe.

Rosemary Roasted Root Vegetables with Kale

ANASTASIA ST. JOHN | COMPASSIONATE DIET AND LIFESTYLE ADVOCATE

KALE IS A delicious and nutritious way to dress up roasted root veggies!

SERVES 6

1 large potato, cut into large cubes
1 carrot, cut into large slices
1 turnip, peeled and cut into cubes
1 medium onion, cut into large wedges
4 garlic cloves, cut in half
¼ teaspoon black pepper
¼ teaspoon chile powder
1 tablespoon rosemary
¾ teaspoon sea salt
2 cups water
2 cups chopped kale

1. Preheat oven to 375°F.
2. Put the potato, carrot, turnip, onion, garlic, black pepper, chile powder, rosemary, and ½ teaspoon of the salt into a large bowl and toss well. Dump the vegetable mixture onto a shallow baking pan, add 1 cup of the water, and bake until the vegetables are soft and their edges are browned, about 45 minutes to 1 hour. While they are cooking, turn the vegetables over once or twice with a spatula. Add more water to the baking pan if needed.
3. Add the remaining 1 cup water to a medium saucepan and bring to a boil. Add the kale and the remaining ¼ teaspoon salt and cover. Reduce heat and steam the kale until soft, about 3 to 5 minutes. Drain the kale, toss with the roasted vegetables, and serve.

MVP (Most Valuable Pesto) Stuffed Mushrooms

CHEF AJ | *UNPROCESSED*

THE FIRST TIME Rip Esselstyn ate at my house he ate twelve of these all by himself! They also got rave reviews from Ann Crile Esselstyn, who had eight.

MAKES 12 STUFFED MUSHROOMS

> **12 cremini mushrooms**
> **1 cup pine nuts**
> **2 garlic cloves (or more to taste)**
> **1 tablespoon low-sodium yellow miso paste**
> **1 cup fresh basil (about 2 ounces)**
> **Juice of 1 lemon**

Remove the stems from the mushrooms and set aside. Put the pine nuts, garlic, miso, basil, and lemon juice into a food processor fitted with the "S" blade and puree until smooth. Fill the mushroom cups with the pine nut mixture and put in a dehydrator. Dehydrate for 2 to 4 hours until warm.

TIP ▶ Removing some of the center of the mushrooms will help you fit more stuffing inside.

TIP ▶ If you don't have a dehydrator, bake the mushrooms at 350°F for an hour, or until soft.

VARIATION:

▶ I like to add about 3 ounces of baby spinach to the mixture for extra nutrition. If you do, be careful: spinach will add water when it heats up, so don't add much and maybe omit the basil.

Maple-Glazed Brussels Sprouts

CHEF AJ | *UNPROCESSED*

EVEN PEOPLE WHO say that they don't normally like Brussels sprouts will enjoy this dish. I like to double the sauce!!!

SERVES 6 TO 8

1½ pound Brussels sprouts

¼ cup finely minced shallots

¼ cup maple syrup

1 tablespoon Dijon mustard

1 tablespoon tamari

1 tablespoon arrowroot powder

Finely diced red bell pepper, optional

Chopped walnuts or pecans, optional

1. Bring a saucepan of water to a boil. Cut the stems off the Brussels sprouts and discard, then cut the sprouts in half. Cook the sprouts in the boiling water for 2 minutes; drain. Rinse with cold water.
2. In heavy nonstick sauce pan, sauté the shallots in a small amount of water or vegetable for 2 to 3 minutes. Add the boiled Brussels sprouts and sauté for 4 more minutes. Whisk together the maple syrup, Dijon mustard, tamari, and arrowroot powder in a small bowl. Pour the maple syrup mixture over the Brussels sprouts and cook for about 2 minutes, until the sauce thickens. Garnish with bell pepper or nuts if desired.

TIP ▶ The first step of cooking and cooling the Brussels sprouts can be done in advance.

Broiled New Potato Puffs

ANN CRILE ESSELSTYN

THESE ARE RIDICULOUSLY easy and ridiculously delicious. They work as well if you just cut the potatoes and put them in the oven with no other preparation. Sweet potatoes work, too.

These are good plain, or try with hummus, ketchup, or salsa.

SERVES 2 TO 4

10 small red potatoes (2 to 3 inches long), sliced into halves or thirds
¼ cup vegetable broth
1 teaspoon rosemary
1 teaspoon lemon pepper

Set oven to broil. Put cut potatoes into a bowl and sprinkle with broth, rosemary, and lemon pepper. Arrange the potatoes in a single layer on a baking sheet and put into the oven, about 8 inches below the broiler. Cook for 15 minutes. Keep peeking to make sure they don't burn. They will puff up and the tops will brown. It is not necessary to flip them over.

Red Potatoes with Kale

KAREN CAMPBELL AND LEANNE CAMPBELL DISLA | *WHOLE PLANTS COOKBOOK*

COLLARD GREENS CAN substitute nicely for the kale in this recipe.

MAKES 6 CUPS

> **4 red potatoes**
> **1 bunch of kale**
> **4 tablespoons water**
> **1 onion, thinly sliced**
> **2 garlic cloves, minced**
> **1 teaspoon sesame seeds**
> **½ teaspoon black pepper**
> **½ teaspoon paprika**
> **2 tablespoons tamari**

1. Scrub the potatoes and cut into ½-inch cubes or wedges. Steam over boiling water until just tender when pierced with a fork. Rinse with cold water, then drain and set aside.
2. Rinse the kale and remove the stems. Cut or tear the leaves into small pieces and set aside.
3. Heat 2 tablespoons of the water in a large nonstick skillet and add the onion, garlic, and sesame seeds. Sauté 5 minutes. Add the cooked potatoes, black pepper, and paprika. Continue cooking until the potatoes begin to brown, about 5 minutes. Use a spatula to turn the mixture gently as it cooks.
4. Spread the kale leaves over the top of the potato mixture. Sprinkle with the remaining 2 tablespoons of water and the tamari. Cover and cook, turning occasionally and adding water as needed, until the kale is tender, about 15 to 20 minutes.

Sweet Potato Fries

RIP ESSELSTYN | *THE ENGINE 2 DIET*

WE LOVE SWEET potato fries at Station 2. Nothing could be easier. We leave the skin on for maximum nutrients and flavor. Sweet potatoes, with their golden orange color, are a rich and vibrant source of beta carotene—hence the bold, carrot-like color.

SERVES 4

2 sweet potatoes with skins on, scrubbed and sliced into strips

Preheat oven to 450°F. Place the potato slices on a sprayed baking sheet and cover with aluminum foil. Cook for 30 to 40 minutes, turning once. Remove the foil after 20 minutes to allow the slices to brown. The thinner your slices, the faster they cook. They are most delicious when lightly brown—but take care not to burn them.

Maple Mashed Sweet Potatoes

MARY MCDOUGALL | THE MCDOUGALL PROGRAM

THIS DISH IS always on our table for our Thanksgiving dinner. I usually make it with garnet yams for the bright orange color and a more creamy consistency.

SERVES 6

> **3 pounds yams**
> **½ cup soy milk**
> **1 tablespoon pure maple syrup**
> **Salt**
> **Freshly ground pepper**

1. Preheat oven to 400°F. Scrub the yams and prick all over with a fork. Place on a baking sheet and bake for about 45 minutes, or until tender. Allow to cool slightly.
2. Cut the yams in half lengthwise and scoop the flesh into a large bowl. Mash with a hand masher or electric beater (do not use a food processor). Add the soy milk and maple syrup; mix well. Add salt and pepper to taste.

TIP ▶ This can be prepared a day or two ahead and refrigerated. Reheat in a microwave before serving. The yams may also be peeled and cooked in boiling water instead of baked. Drain off the cooking water, allow to cool slightly, and proceed as above.

Just Potatoes? Potatoes

SAN'DERA PRUDE | FEATURED IN *FORKS OVER KNIVES*

PEOPLE COME TO my house and ask me, What are you cooking in there? Potatoes? It smells like you're cooking meat up in here!

Herbs can be fresh or dried, whatever you have on hand.

Potatoes, diced
Onions, diced
White pepper
Parsley
Thyme
Dry mustard
Cayenne

Put the potatoes in a sauté pan with a little water and the onions. Sprinkle with the pepper, parsley, thyme, mustard, cayenne, and oregano. Cover and cook over low-medium heat until the potatoes are soft. Adjust the seasonings to taste. Let the odor fill your house.

Potato Salad

ALAN GOLDHAMER AND DOUG LISLE | *THE HEALTH PROMOTING COOKBOOK*

COMFORT FOOD WITHOUT the fat—this is a favorite of our patients. The flavors improve with time. This goes well with a green salad and or as a complement to other salad dishes.

SERVES 8

> **12 cups red creamer potatoes, cut into 1-inch cubes**
> **1 cup celery juice or vegetable stock**
> **3 cups water**
> **3 ribs celery, diced**
> **2 carrots, diced**
> **1 red or green bell pepper, diced**
> **½ cup diced green onions**
> **1½ tablespoons dill weed**
> **1 teaspoon basil**
> **½ teaspoon garlic powder**
> **½ teaspoon onion powder**

In a 4-quart saucepan, simmer the potatoes in the juice or stock and water until just tender. Allow to cool. In a large mixing bowl, combine the remaining ingredients, and let stand to marry the flavors. When the ingredients are cool, mix all the ingredients together, and serve.

Lovely Collard Wraps with Red Pepper and Cucumber

ANN CRILE ESSELSTYN

THESE ARE STUNNING—BOTH beautiful and delicious—and so much fun to make, they don't feel like work. For the filling, substitute cooked asparagus or green beans; long, thinly sliced carrot or bok choy strips; cooked greens; or rice and beans. ANYTHING is good in them. They make perfect sushi-like hors d'oeuvres, or eat them instead of sandwiches.

1 bunch of collards

½ cup oil-free, no-tahini hummus

2 green onions, chopped

½ cup fresh cilantro, chopped

¼ cup shredded carrots

¼ red bell pepper, cut into thin strips

¼ small cucumber, cut into thin strips (skin optional)

½ lemon

1. Put about 2 inches of water in a large sauté pan and bring to a boil.
2. Choose 4 of the nicest collard leaves. Lay them flat, cut off the thick stem at the point where the leaf begins, then place them into the boiling water, one on top of the other. Cover and cook for 30 seconds to 1 minute; drain.
3. Lay a cooked collard leaf flat on a board or counter with the thick part of the stem facing up and running horizontally. Put a row of about 2 tablespoons hummus below and along the center spine, then sprinkle the hummus with green onions, cilantro, and shredded carrots. Place bell pepper strips and cucumber strips, running horizontally, on top.
4. Fold the edge of the leaf nearest you over the filling and gently roll the leaf around the filling and into a sausage shape. With a sharp knife, cut the roll into as many *small* round pieces as possible. You should be able to get six or more pieces, but it will depend on the size of your leaf. The creator always gets to eat the end pieces!

TIP ▶ Collards are pretty tough and don't easily break apart when cooked. Their flexibility makes them a perfect wrap!

Quinoa and Kale Stuffed Tomato

MOIRA NORDHOLT | THE FEEL GOOD GURU

THIS DISH LOOKS elegant on a plate and is a beautiful, light, and healthy meal to serve to guests. This recipe serves one—for more, simply cook more quinoa, and "eyeball" additional veggies to create a nice mixture.

SERVES 1

> 1 cup quinoa
> 2 cups water or unsalted vegetable broth
> Himalayan sea salt
> 3 garlic cloves, minced
> ¼ red onion, finely diced
> ½ cup of broccoli florets
> 4 dinosaur kale leaves, cut into fine ribbons
> Tamari
> 1 large organic heirloom tomato, cored
> Juice of 1 lemon

1. Rinse the quinoa well and drain in a fine sieve. Put in a saucepan with the water and salt, bring to a boil, then reduce the heat and simmer for 10 to 15 minutes until all the water is absorbed.
2. In a large cast iron frying pan, heat a splash of spring water or broth and sauté garlic, onion, broccoli, and kale. When the broccoli and kale have turned dark green, add a splash of tamari and stir. Remove from heat.
3. When the quinoa is cooked, add some of it to the vegetable mixture and combine well. (You decide how much.) Hollow out the center of the tomato and fill with the quinoa-vegetable mixture.
4. Serve the stuffed tomato with the rest of the vegetable-quinoa mixture on the side, and drizzle with a squeeze of fresh lemon to make the flavors pop!

VARIATION:

▶ The stuffed tomato can be warmed in a hot oven for 10 minutes or until heated through.

Squash Pudding

JO STEPANIAK | *BREAKING THE FOOD SEDUCTION* BY NEAL BARNARD, MD

MASHED WINTER SQUASH is a sweet and colorful alternative to ordinary mashed potatoes. It's also the perfect holiday side dish in place of yams, and it even makes a tasty dessert, especially if you add a few toasted, chopped pecans.

SERVES 4

4 cups peeled butternut squash cut into cubes
3 tablespoons pure maple syrup
2 tablespoons sesame tahini, peanut butter, or almond butter
½ teaspoon vanilla extract
Salt

Steam squash cubes until very soft. Transfer to a food processor along with the remaining ingredients and process until very smooth. Season with salt to taste. Serve hot.

Easy Cranberry Relish

CHEF AJ | *UNPROCESSED*

WHY COOK YOUR relish or use sugar when you can make this instead?

2 large oranges
One 12-ounce bag fresh cranberries
Date syrup, optional

Zest the oranges, then peel and discard rinds. Put the zest, peeled oranges, and cranberries into a food processor fitted with the "S" blade and pulse until a nice chunky texture. If you want a sweeter relish, add a bit of date syrup.

VARIATION:

▶ Substitute fresh ginger and lime juice for the oranges and orange zest for a delicious variation.

Cauliflower Rice

DARSHANA THACKER | AYURVEDIC VEGAN CHEF

THIS IS A twist on basic steamed rice. The flavor from the cauliflower and spices is so subtle that it complements any kind of lentil or vegetable dishes, including dal.

SERVES 4 TO 6

> **1 cup rice (preferably basmati)**
> **2 cups water**
> **½ teaspoon cumin seeds**
> **½ teaspoon grated fresh ginger**
> **¼ teaspoon green chile paste**
> **1 cup finely chopped cauliflower**
> **½ teaspoon salt**
> **1 tablespoon finely chopped cilantro**

1. Wash the rice, changing the water at least 3 times. Put the rice and water into a saucepan and bring to a boil. Reduce the heat, cover, and cook for 10 minutes. Set aside.
2. Roast the cumin seeds lightly in a skillet for about 1 to 2 minutes. Add the ginger and chile paste; stir. Add the cauliflower, cooked rice, and salt. Cook for 2 to 3 minutes. Garnish with cilantro.

Garlic Rosemary Polenta

MICAELA COOK | T. COLIN CAMPBELL FOUNDATION

WHEN I CUT back on eating bread, polenta became one of my favorite foods. Served with pinto beans, greens, and baked onions, it makes a most satisfying healthy meal.

SERVES 6

> 1 medium onion, finely chopped
>
> 3 cloves minced garlic
>
> 2 tablespoons rosemary, ground if possible
>
> 1 teaspoon salt, or to taste
>
> 2 cups dry corn grits
>
> 3 cups vegetable broth
>
> 2 cups unflavored plant-based milk (see page 68)
>
> ⅓ cup chopped sundried tomatoes, optional, for extra flavor

1. Preheat the oven to 350°F.
2. Mix together the onion, garlic, rosemary, salt, and corn grits. Add the broth and plant milk.
3. Bring to a boil in pot, turn down to a simmer, and stir gently until mixture is thick, about 10 minutes. Pour into a pie pan and bake for 30 minutes.

> **TIP ▶** If you are out of broth or plant milk you can also use water; it may not be quite as flavorful, but it still works.

Sensational Herbed Bread

LEANNE CAMPBELL DISLA | *WHOLE PLANTS COOKBOOK*

THIS TASTY AND savory bread is a perfect side with soup, pasta, or salad or as a snack. It takes a quick 15 minutes to prepare, and you only need to let the bread rise once, which makes it easy. If you want plain bread, simply omit the herbs—it's just as delicious!

MAKES 1 LOAF

- 3 cups whole wheat flour
- ½ tablespoon sage
- ½ tablespoon thyme
- ½ tablespoon basil
- ½ tablespoon oregano
- 1½ teaspoons dry yeast
- 2 teaspoon molasses
- 1¾ cups lukewarm water

1. Line a 9 × 5-inch bread pan with parchment paper. Set aside. Combine the flour, sage, thyme, basil, and oregano in a large mixing bowl. Stir in the yeast. Make a well in the center of the flour and pour in the molasses and water. Mix by hand to make a soft, slightly wet dough. Knead until the dough leaves the sides of the bowl clean and feels elastic.
2. Preheat oven to 400°F. Place the dough in the pan, cover with oiled plastic wrap, and leave in a warm, draft-free place until doubled in size, about 1 hour. Bake for about 35 minutes. Test to see if the bread is ready by tapping the top with your knuckles: the bread is done when it sounds hollow.

VARIATION:

▶ Fresh herbs can also be used in this recipe, and for a slightly different taste, rosemary and chives can be substituted for the thyme and basil.

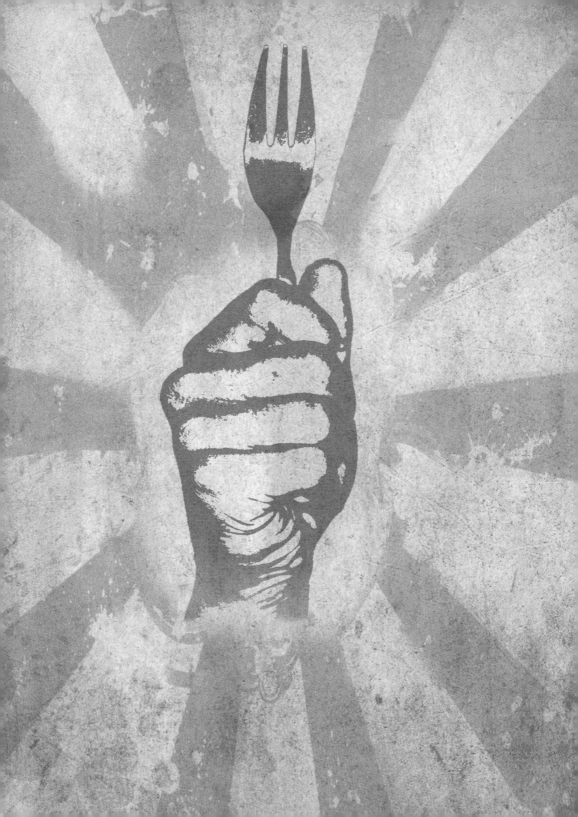

Fruit with Lime, Mint, and Orange Juice

ANN CRILE ESSELSTYN | *PREVENT AND REVERSE HEART DISEASE*

HERE, THE ADDITION of orange juice, lime juice with zest, and mint transcends cut-up fruit into a special dessert to use all year round. Everyone always asks, "What is in this?" It is GOOD!

You can make this with any fruit you have available.

SERVES 6 TO 8

Cantaloupe and/or honeydew
Strawberries, sliced
Blueberries and/or raspberries
Orange sections
Kiwi, sliced
Orange juice
Zest and juice of ½ lime
Fresh mint

Cut the melon into ½-inch pieces or use a melon baller. Put into a bowl, add strawberries, blueberries, orange sections, and kiwi, and toss gently. Add enough orange juice to partially cover the fruit. Sprinkle with the lime zest and juice and stir in the mint leaves.

DESSERTS

Baked Stuffed Apples

LEWIS FREEDMAN AND PRISCILLA TIMBERLAKE | *COMMUNITY DINNERS SERVED WITH LOVE*

EVERY BITE OF this dessert is filled with flavor. It's a wonderful autumn treat that can substitute for traditional pie.

SERVES 8

¼ **cup seedless raisins**
¼ **cup roasted walnuts, chopped**
1½ **teaspoons dark miso**
½ **cup tahini**
½ **cup rice syrup**
1 **teaspoon cinnamon**
⅓ **cup water**
8 **baking apples**
1 **cup apple juice**

1. Preheat oven to 375°F.
2. Mix together the raisins, walnuts, miso, tahini, rice syrup, cinnamon, and water in a small bowl. Core the apples, but not all the way through: leave enough at the bottom to hold the filling. Stuff each apple with the tahini mixture. Place stuffed apples in a small baking dish and pour the apple juice into the pan and over the apples. Bake for 1 hour or more, depending on the apple variety.

Banana Ice Cream

MARY MCDOUGALL | THE MCDOUGALL PROGRAM

THIS FROZEN DESSERT requires frozen bananas, which can also make a delicious addition to smoothies. When you have extra ripe bananas, peel them, break them into pieces, place them in a freezer bag, and freeze for at least 1 day.

6 frozen bananas
1 tablespoon vanilla
½ cup soy or almond milk

Puree a few of the frozen banana pieces, about a teaspoon of the vanilla, and a small amount of the milk in a food processor until smooth. Pour into a large bowl, then repeat this step until all the bananas are processed. Quickly stir the "ice cream," and serve at once.

VARIATION:

▶ Other frozen fruits may be added along with the frozen bananas for additional flavor.

Frozen Chocolate Banana Treats

ANN CRILE ESSELSTYN | THE ESSELSTYN FAMILY

TIFF CUNNINGHAM, OUR daughter-in-law's sister, sent us the idea for this recipe, and we think it is the healthiest, most decadent-tasting dessert we have had in a long time. Be sure to serve these frozen. This recipe makes about fifty, depending on how many you eat as you go. Even if you eat them all, it isn't so awful!

Rolling the balls in Grape-Nuts keeps the chocolate from melting on your fingers when you eat these. Kashi 7 Whole Grain Nuggets are especially crunchy, but anything like Grape-Nuts will work. These are wonderful without Grape-Nuts, too, just messy.

MAKES ABOUT 50

⅓ cup maple syrup
⅓ cup plant-based milk (see page 68)
⅓ cup cocoa powder
2 teaspoons vanilla
2 ripe bananas
2 cups oats
Grape-Nuts

1. Puree the maple syrup, milk, cocoa, vanilla, and bananas in a food processor until well combined. Transfer to a bowl. Add the oats and mix well.

2. Line a baking sheet with wax paper. Put Grape-Nuts in a small bowl. Using the big end of a melon baller or a small spoon, scoop up a little chocolate ball and drop it into the bowl of Grape-Nuts. Turn the ball over with a spoon or your fingers (you may find it easiest to use your fingers), then sprinkle Grape-Nuts onto the sides and gently place it onto the wax paper. I like to flatten the ball a little with the back of a spoon. Repeat this process with the rest of the chocolate mixture.

3. Freeze the entire pan of chocolate treats. After the treats are frozen, transfer them to an airtight container and store it in the freezer. Actually, hide it so you can't see it easily!

Instant Chocolate Pudding

JO STEPANIAK | *BREAKING THE FOOD SEDUCTION* BY NEAL BARNARD, MD

GREAT HOMEMADE CHOCOLATE pudding in under five minutes? You bet! You'll be an instant believer with this remarkable recipe.

MAKES ABOUT 1¾ CUPS

> 1½ cups (about 12 ounces) firm silken tofu, crumbled
> ¼ to ½ cup dry sweetener or pure maple syrup
> ⅓ cup unsweetened cocoa or carob powder
> 2 teaspoons vanilla extract
> Pinch of salt, optional

Place all ingredients in food processor and blend several minutes until smooth and creamy. Chill in the refrigerator until serving time.

TIP ▶ Start with the smaller amount of sweetener and add a little more, as needed to suit your taste.

Lime Mousse

ANN CRILE ESSELSTYN

THIS IS DELICIOUS alone, topped with fruit of any kind, or as a frosting on cake. It is fast to make at the last minute. Use more or less lime according to taste. It is especially beautiful in a wineglass with fresh raspberries and sprinkled with mint. Be sure to use SILKEN tofu.

SERVES 2 TO 4

> **One 12.3-ounce package Mori-Nu Silken Lite Firm or Extra Firm tofu**
> **⅓ cup maple syrup or sweetener of choice**
> **3 tablespoons fresh lime juice**
> **Zest of 1 lime**

Puree the tofu, maple syrup, and lime juice and zest in a food processor until very smooth. Keep scraping down the sides of the processor to blend completely. Refrigerate until chilled.

Oatmeal-Raisin Cookies

ADAPTED FROM ALAN GOLDHAMER AND DOUG LISLE | *THE HEALTH PROMOTING COOKBOOK*

MOIST AND DELICIOUS, these cookies are a sweet and satisfying snack or dessert. Don't be fooled by their wet appearance when you take them out of the oven—they'll harden slightly when cool, but they ARE cooked and ready to eat.

SERVES 12 | MAKES 24 COOKIES

> **4 cups oats ground in a food processor or coffee grinder**
> **1 teaspoon baking powder**
> **½ teaspoon baking soda**
> **1 teaspoon cinnamon**
> **¼ teaspoon nutmeg**
> **2 large ripe bananas, mashed**
> **1 cup apple juice**
> **½ cup raisins**

Preheat the oven to 375°F. Mix the dry ingredients in a large bowl. In a food processor, blend the bananas and juice until smooth. Slowly add the dry ingredients while mixing. Pour the batter into the large bowl, and add the raisins. Drop by spoonfuls onto a nonstick baking sheet. Press down with the bottom of a glass to flatten. Bake for 10 minutes.

Fast Cookies for School Lunches

KAREN CAMPBELL | THE CAMPBELL FAMILY

THESE EASY SNACKS are a hit with young and old alike.

MAKES ABOUT 8 COOKIES

⅓ cup maple syrup

⅓ cup almond milk

¼ cup cocoa

3 tablespoons peanut butter

1 teaspoon vanilla

1½ cups oats

¼ cup walnuts, optional

Put maple syrup, almond milk, and cocoa into a saucepan, bring to a boil, then simmer for 3 minutes. Add the peanut butter and stir until dissolved. Remove from the heat and add the vanilla, oats, and walnuts. Stir well, then form into small cookies.

Outrageous Brownies

CHEF AJ | AUTHOR OF *UNPROCESSED*

THESE BROWNIES ARE like the friend you can bring to any party—they get along with everyone.

MAKES 8 BROWNIES

One 15-ounce can salt-free black beans, drained and rinsed

1½ cups date syrup

2 tablespoons ground flax seeds

1 tablespoon alcohol-free vanilla extract

½ teaspoon caramel extract

1 teaspoon baking powder

½ teaspoon baking soda

½ cup raw cocoa (Ultimate SuperFoods is my favorite brand)

¾ cup barley flour

1 cup Sunspire nondairy grain-sweetened chocolate chips

Preheat oven to 350°F. Put beans and date syrup into the bowl of a food processor fitted with the "S" blade and process until smooth. Add the flax seeds, vanilla and caramel extracts, baking powder, baking soda, and cocoa and process again. Add the flour and pulse until just combined. Stir in the chocolate chips. Pour the batter into an 8 × 8-inch square silicone baking pan. Bake for 30 to 35 minutes until the middle does not jiggle and a toothpick inserted into it comes out clean.

Crispy Rice Bars

JO STEPANIAK | *BREAKING THE FOOD SEDUCTION* BY NEAL BARNARD, MD

THESE CRUNCHY, NUTTY squares make a delicious dessert or sweet snack.

MAKES 16 SQUARES

⅔ cup brown rice syrup

¼ cup natural almond butter or peanut butter

½ teaspoon vanilla extract

2 cups crisped rice cereal

ADDITIONS (CHOOSE ONE)

½ cup lightly roasted chopped almonds or walnuts

½ cup currants, raisins, or finely chopped apricots

½ cup nondairy carob chips

1. Mist an 8-inch square pan with nonstick cooking spray and set aside.
2. Place the brown rice syrup and nut butter in a small saucepan and warm until the mixture is softened and smooth. Remove from the heat and stir in vanilla extract. Combine the cereal and the addition of your choice in a large bowl. Pour the warm mixture over the cereal mix and combine carefully, using a wooden spoon. Work as quickly as possible (this is especially important if using carob chips so they do not melt). Pack the mixture evenly into the prepared pan, pressing gently with your fingers. Cover with plastic wrap and chill until firm. Slice into squares and store in an airtight container in the refrigerator.

Raw Date Power Bars

MOIRA NORDHOLT | THE FEEL GOOD GURU

THESE RAW DATE squares are a powerful way to start the day, a perfect food to grab either before or after a workout or a hike or just about any time you need an energy boost or a pick-me-up between meals. They're simple to whip up in a food processor in five minutes and ready to eat immediately. They won't last long once they're sitting out on the counter, but if you're able to ration, they'll improve with a little rest in the fridge or an overnight on the countertop. These quantities are for a small baking pan.

SERVES 8 TO 10

> **1 cup fresh or dried dates, pitted**
> **1½ cup organic almonds**
> **1 banana**
> **½ cup cacao nibs**
> **1 teaspoon vanilla extract**
> **Dried shredded coconut**

1. If using dried dates, soak them for a few minutes in just enough water or orange juice to cover; drain.
2. Pulse the almonds in a dry food processor until they're broken up but still in crunchy chunks. Add the banana, cocoa nibs, and vanilla and blend just until mixed.
3. Sprinkle coconut over the bottom of a small square baking pan. Scrape the mixture onto the pan and spread it out evenly; press it down gently with your hands. Sprinkle coconut over the top.
4. An hour or more of refrigeration will make it easier to cut into bars and serve, but these are at their gooey, datey, tasty best at room temperature.

Pear-Cranberry Crumble

MARY MCDOUGALL | THE MCDOUGALL PROGRAM

I HAD SOME fresh cranberries in my refrigerator that my grandson, Jaysen, wanted to use. I also had fresh pears, so we decided to make a dessert. While it was cooling on the rack, everyone came in for a sample, and we all decided it was a hit!

SERVES 8 TO 10

THE TOPPING

> ½ cup rolled oats
>
> ½ cup chopped walnuts
>
> ¼ cup white whole wheat flour
>
> ½ teaspoon cinnamon
>
> ¼ teaspoon nutmeg
>
> 2 tablespoons agave nectar

THE FILLING:

> 3 cups peeled, cubed Bosc pears
>
> 2 cups fresh cranberries
>
> ⅓ cup brown sugar
>
> 2½ tablespoons cornstarch

1. Preheat oven to 350°F.
2. For the topping, combine the oats, walnuts, flour, cinnamon, and nutmeg in a medium bowl and mix well, then add agave nectar and mix until crumbled. Set aside.
3. For the filling, combine all the filling ingredients in a large bowl; mix well.
4. Transfer the pear mixture into to a deep-dish pie plate and sprinkle the topping mixture over the top. Bake for about 1 hour, until the filling is bubbly and the top is lightly browned. Cool for 1 hour before serving (if you can wait!).

TIP ► I used Bosc pears because they tend to keep their shape when cooked and don't get too mushy.

VARIATION:

► When fresh cranberries are not available, frozen, thawed berries may be used in their place. This is also delicious made with apples and blueberries.

Raspberry-Pear Crisp

CHEF DEL SROUFE | WELLNESS FORUM FOODS

CINNAMON-SPICED PEARS AND fresh raspberries baked under a crunchy oat topping will make this healthy dessert a classic in your kitchen. If you would like, substitute blueberries for the raspberries, which will make this an appealing dish you can serve any time of the year.

SERVES 6

FILLING

> 7 fresh pears, cut into ½-inch dice
>
> ½ cup maple syrup
>
> ¾ teaspoon stevia powder (a healthy, all-natural alternative to sugar)
>
> ¼ teaspoon sea salt, optional
>
> 1 teaspoon cinnamon
>
> Pinch of nutmeg
>
> 1 pint fresh raspberries

TOPPING

> 1½ cups rolled oats
>
> ½ cup maple syrup
>
> ½ cup apple juice
>
> ½ teaspoon cinnamon
>
> Pinch of sea salt, optional

1. Preheat oven to 375°F.
2. For the filling: Combine the pears and maple syrup in a large saucepan. Cook over medium heat, covered but stirring occasionally, until the pears are tender, about 10 to 12 minutes. Remove the pears from the heat and add the stevia, sea salt, cinnamon, and nutmeg. Transfer the filling into a 9 × 13-inch baking pan. Sprinkle with the fresh raspberries.
3. For the topping: Combine all the topping ingredients and spread over the filling.
4. Bake for 25 to 30 minutes.

Fruit Pie with Date-Nut Crust

RIP ESSELSTYN | *THE ENGINE 2 DIET*

THIS FABULOUS PIE was given to us by Austin singer and songwriter Libby Fitzpatrick shortly after our son Kole was born. It is sinfully simple and succulently delicious.

SERVES 4 TO 6

CRUST

1 cup dates

⅓ cup walnuts

⅓ cup cashews

⅓ cup almonds

1 teaspoon vanilla extract

FILLING

2 to 3 bananas, sliced lengthwise

4 ounces strawberries, sliced

4 ounces strawberries, blended into a puree

4 ounces raspberries

1 can Mandarin oranges, drained

Blend the crust ingredients together in a food processor to achieve a sticky consistency. Press the blended crust ingredients into a pie pan. Lay the bananas on top of the crust and press along the sides. Place the strawberry slices on top of the bananas. Pour the strawberry puree over the strawberries and bananas, and press into the gaps. Place the raspberries and Mandarin oranges on top of the pie. Cover and refrigerate for 1 hour before serving.

Fresh Strawberry Pie

LEANNE CAMPBELL DISLA | *WHOLE PLANTS COOKBOOK*

THIS PIE ALWAYS gets rave reviews, even from people used to sugary desserts. Serve with a sprig of mint for decoration, and people will be asking for seconds and thirds.

SERVES 8

> **2 cups low-fat crushed graham crackers**
> **½ cup apple juice**
> **1½ cups sliced fresh strawberries**
> **¾ cup water**
> **1 cup frozen or fresh whole strawberries**
> **¼ cup cornstarch**
> **⅓ cup dry sweetener**

1. Crush the graham crackers into a medium bowl and mix with the apple juice. Press the mixture into a 9-inch pie pan. Arrange sliced strawberries in an even layer, over the graham cracker crust. Set aside.
2. Bring the water and whole strawberries to a boil in a medium saucepan until strawberries start to dissolve. Mix together the cornstarch and dry sweetener in a small bowl and add to boiling strawberries; stir well. Cook over medium-low heat until the mixture thickens, stirring constantly for 3 to 4 minutes. Once the mixture is thick, pour it over the sliced strawberries in the pie dish. Refrigerate for 2 to 3 hours before serving.

VARIATION:

▶ Other fruits can be used in place of strawberries. Both blueberries and peaches work well in this recipe.

Cherry Pineapple Cake

KAREN CAMPBELL | THE CAMPBELL FAMILY

THIS CAKE MELTS in your mouth, and the visual effect is quite beautiful.

SERVES 8 TO 10

FRUIT MIXTURE

- 1 can red tart cherries
- 1 can crushed pineapple
- ½ cup unsweetened shredded coconut
- ½ cup sweetener, such as maple powder or honey
- ½ cup chopped walnuts, optional

TOPPING

- 1½ cups whole wheat flour
- ½ cup oat flour
- 1½ teaspoons baking powder
- ¼ cup sweetener, such as maple powder
- 1½ cups plant-based milk (I like almond milk; see page 68)

1. Preheat the oven to 350°F. For the fruit mixture, combine the cherries, pineapple, coconut, sweetener, and walnuts in a 9 × 13-inch baking pan. Spread out evenly.
2. For the topping, combine the wheat flour, oat flour, baking powder, sweetener, and milk in a small bowl and pour it over the fruit mixture. Do not stir.
3. Bake at 350°F for 45 to 50 minutes.

Sexy Raw Carrot Cake

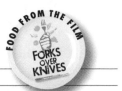

MOIRA NORDHOLT | THE FEEL GOOD GURU

THIS BEAUTIFUL CAKE has all the flavor and decadence of a traditional carrot cake without the refined flour, oil, eggs, icing sugar, and cream cheese!

Remember, there's no flour holding this cake together. Extracting the carrot cake in nice wedges requires an angel's touch.

SERVES 6

> 1 cup organic raisins
> 1 large or 2 medium carrots, finely grated
> 2 cups whole walnuts, chopped finely
> ½ cup organic shredded coconut
> 1 tablespoon tahini
> ¼ cup maple syrup (or less—usually just a splash will do)
> 1 teaspoon vanilla extract
> Pinch of cinnamon
> Pinch of nutmeg
> Pinch of cloves
> Vegan "Cream Cheese" Icing (page 196)

1. Soak the raisins in spring water until plump, then rinse and finely chop. Put into a large bowl and add the carrots, walnuts, coconut, tahini, maple syrup, vanilla, cinnamon, nutmeg, and cloves. Mix well, then press the mixture firmly into a small round pan or glass pie dish.
2. Let sit for at least 1 hour. Frost with Vegan "Cream Cheese" Icing and serve.

Vegan "Cream Cheese" Icing

MOIRA NORDHOLT | THE FEEL GOOD GURU

THIS RICH AND creamy topping is perfect on more than just carrot cake, and even people used to sugar and butter will love it.

MAKES ENOUGH FOR ONE CAKE

> **1 cup cashews**
> **Juice from 1 lemon**
> **⅛ to ¼ cup maple syrup**
> **1 teaspoon pure vanilla extract**

Puree the cashews, lemon juice, maple syrup, vanilla extract, and a splash of water in a blender at high speed to create a smooth, creamy, thick consistency, then spread or pour over cake.

TIP ▶ Try blending the cashews first with just the lemon juice and maple syrup, then add water a splash at a time as needed to achieve the desired consistency. A powerful Vitamix blender on high speed is able to make a silky, creamy texture. If you soak the cashews overnight and then drain them, you won't need to add any water.

CONVERSION CHARTS

FRUITS		
Blackberries	1 cup	115 g
Blueberries	1 cup	110 g
Cranberries	1 cup	170 g
Currants	½ cup	80 g
Dates, pitted	1 cup	160 g
Raisins	1 cup	160 g
Strawberries	1 cup	150 g

VEGETABLES		
Arugula	1 cup	70 g
Basil	1 cup	57 g
Broccoli florets	1 cup	85 g
Brussels sprouts	1½ pounds	680 g
Cabbage, shredded	1 cup	60 g
Cauliflower	1 cup florets	85 g
Cilantro, chopped	½ cup	10 g
Eggplant	1 medium	340 g
Parsley	1 small bunch	60 g
Peas	⅓ cup	44 g
Mushrooms	6 ounces	170 g
Spinach	1 cup	70 g
Yam	1 medium	340 g

BEANS		
Black beans, cooked	½ cup	130 g
Chickpeas, cooked	1 cup	260 g
Lentils, dry	1 cup	200 g
Polenta/grits	1 cup	140 g
Tofu, firm	14 ounces	395 g
Tofu, silken	12.3 ounces	344 g
White beans, dry	1 cup	180 g

GRAINS		
Pearl barley, dry	½ cup	88 g
Quinoa	1 cup	185 g
Rice	1 cup	200 g
Rolled oats	1 cup	205 g

FLOURS		
Cocoa powder	¼ cup	25 g
Cornstarch	2 tablespoons	17 g
Flaxseed meal	1 tablespoon	7 g
Nutritional yeast	1 tablespoon	5 g
Oat flour	½ cup	45 g
Whole-wheat flour	1 cup	140 g

NUTS AND SEEDS		
Almonds	½ cup	65 g
Cashews, whole	½ cup	75 g
Hemp seeds	2 tablespoons	15 g
Peanuts	½ cup	75 g
Pecans, halved	½ cup	50 g
Pine nuts	¼ cup	30 g
Pistachios, shelled	½ cup	70 g
Sesame seeds	½ cup	35 g
Sunflower seeds	½ cup	70 g
Walnuts, halved	½ cup	50 g

SWEETENERS AND FLAVORINGS		
Maple syrup	¼ cup	70 g
Miso paste	1 tablespoon	18 g
Molasses	1 teaspoon	5 g

Appendix

To Learn More

For more information, or to become actively involved in the field of plant-based nutrition, check out these Web sites*:

- ▶ Dr. Neal Barnard's Physician's Committee for Responsible Medicine: www.pcrm.org
- ▶ Gene Baur's Farm Sanctuary site: www.farmsanctuary.org
- ▶ The T. Colin Campbell Foundation, with eCornell, offers a Certificate in Plant-Based Nutrition upon completion of three online courses: www.tcolincampbell.org/courses
- ▶ Dr. Caldwell Esselstyn's *Prevent and Reverse Heart Disease* site: www.heartattackproof.com
- ▶ Rip Esselstyn's *The Engine 2 Diet* site: www.theengine2diet.com
- ▶ Dr. Douglas Graham's site: www.foodnsport.com
- ▶ Dr. Alan Goldhamer's TrueNorth Health Center (where Dr. Doug Lisle is based): www.healthpromoting.com
- ▶ Dr. John McDougall's Immersion Program: www.drmcdougall.com
- ▶ Dr. Pam Popper's Wellness Forum Institute for Health Studies: www.wellnessforuminstitute.org
- ▶ Dr. Alona Pulde and Dr. Matt Lederman's Exsalus Health and Wellness Center: www.exsalus.com

---

* Please note that although URLs are current at time of publication, they are subject to change.

Bookshelf

Some essential books for the plant-based bibliophile:

21-Day Weight-Loss Kickstart by Neal D. Barnard, MD, Grand Central, 2011.

Breaking the Food Seduction by Neal D. Barnard, MD, St. Martin's Press, 2003.

The China Study by T. Colin Campbell, PhD, and Thomas M. Campbell II, BenBella Books, 2006.

Dr. Neal Barnard's Program for Reversing Diabetes by Neal D. Barnard, MD, Rodale, 2007.

The Engine 2 Diet by Rip Esselstyn, Grand Central Books, 2009.

Farm Sanctuary by Gene Baur, Touchstone, 2008.

Foods That Fight Pain by Neal D. Barnard, MD, Harmony/Random House, 1998.

Keep It Simple, Keep It Whole by Alona Pulde, MD, and Matthew Lederman, MD, Exsalus Health & Wellness Center, 2009.

The McDougall Plan for Maximum Weight Loss by John A. McDougall, MD, Plume, 1995.

The McDougall Program for a Healthy Heart by John A. McDougall, MD, Plume 1998.

The McDougall Program: 12 Days to Dynamic Health by John A. McDougall, MD, Plume, 1991.

The McDougall Quick & Easy Cookbook by John A. McDougall, MD, and Mary McDougall, Plume, 1999.

The Pleasure Trap by Douglas J. Lisle, PhD, and Alan Goldhamer, DC, Book Publishing Company, 2006.

Prevent and Reverse Heart Disease by Caldwell B. Esselstyn Jr., MD, Avery Books, 2007.

Solving America's Health Care Crisis by Pam Popper, ND, PB Industries, 2010.

ABOUT THE
RECIPE CONTRIBUTORS

CHEF AJ is the author of the cookbook *Unprocessed* and a culinary instructor and pastry chef at Santé La Brea restaurant in Los Angeles. She has followed a plant-based diet for over thirty-three years.

YOANNAH BROWN is one of the faces behind the delicious menu at Chicago restaurant Soul Vegetarian East, one of Dr. Terry Mason's favorite venues. She follows a vegan lifestyle.

KAREN CAMPBELL was instrumental in inspiring her husband, Dr. Colin Campbell, to write *The China Study* and collaborate on the film *Forks Over Knives*. She has developed hundreds of nourishing, plant-based meals for the Campbell family.

KRIS CARR is the *New York Times* best-selling author of *Crazy Sexy Diet* and the founder of crazysexylife.com. Also a motivational speaker and wellness coach, she wrote and directed the documentary *Crazy Sexy Cancer*.

LEANNE CAMPBELL DISLA, PHD, is the author of the *Whole Plants Cookbook* (www.wholeplantscookbook.com). The daughter of Dr. Colin Campbell, she follows a plant-based diet, along with her sons Steven and Nelson.

MICAELA COOK is the director of the T. Colin Campbell Foundation and a graduate student in nutrition at Johns Hopkins School of Public Health. She enjoys gardening, plant-based cooking, and spending time outdoors with her enthusiastic dog, Chester.

ANN CRILE ESSELSTYN has followed a plant-based diet for more than twenty years, creating original plant-based recipes for herself and her family. She works together with her husband, Dr. Caldwell Esselstyn, to counsel patients at the Cleveland Clinic, and is the author of the recipes in *Prevent and Reverse Heart Disease.*

LEWIS FREEDMAN, a registered dietitian, is an instructor with Dr. Colin Campbell's online certificate program in Plant-Based Nutrition, offered through eCornell. He also teaches yoga and stress management at Cornell. **PRISCILLA TIMBERLAKE** is a whole-foods cook and wellness instructor at Cornell. For over 15 years, they have offered cooking classes and hosted a weekly plant-based dinner in their home. They are currently writing a cookbook, *Community Dinners Served with Love.* They have four children and one daughter-in-law.

RORY FREEDMAN is the coauthor of the nationally bestselling *Skinny Bitch* series of diet books. A former modeling agent with Ford Models, she is out to inspire others to choose healthy foods—and enjoy them!

KATHY FRESTON is the bestselling author of *Quantum Wellness and Veganist.* She promotes a body/mind/spirit approach to health and happiness. She has been featured on *Oprah, Ellen, The Dr. Oz Show, Good Morning America,* and *Extra* and is a regular contributor to *The Huffington Post.*

DR. ALAN GOLDHAMER is a graduate of Western States Chiropractic College in Portland, Oregon, and a licensed chiropractic physician. He is the director of the TrueNorth Health Center, author of *The Health Promoting Cookbook,* and coauthor of *The Pleasure Trap.*

JULIEANNA HEVER, MS, RD, CPT, is known as the Plant-Based Dietitian. She is the executive director of EarthSave, International, the author of the forthcoming *Complete Idiot's Guide to Plant-Based Nutrition,* and *Complete Idiot's Guide to Gluten-Free Vegan Cooking,* a nutrition columnist at *VegNews,* and the coproducer and star of the infotainment documentary *To Your Health.* Visit her at www.toyourhealthnutrition.com.

MARY McDOUGALL, a nurse and educator, has coauthored nine nationally bestselling books with her husband, Dr. John McDougall, including *The McDougall Program.* She oversees the dining component of the McDougall live-in programs and lectures nationwide on practical ways to cook healthy food for the whole family.

ISA CHANDRA MOSKOWITZ is an award-winning vegan chef and author of several best-selling cookbooks, including *Appetite for Reduction and Veganomicon.* A Brooklyn native, she began her vegan cooking journey more than twenty years ago. You can find her cooking and writing at The Post Punk Kitchen (theppk.com).

CHRISTY MORGAN is a "green chick," holistic nutritionist, cooking instructor, and vegan macrobiotic chef in Dallas, Texas. Better known as "The Blissful Chef," she'll show you how to cook food that will make you feel radiant inside and out. Look for her first cookbook, *Blissful Bites*, and more recipes at www .theblissfulchef.com.

ELISE MURPHY works as Creative Director at the T. Colin Campbell Foundation. She lives in Ithaca, NY, with her husband Jack and daughter Sasha. They all eat a plant-based diet.

MOIRA NORDHOLT is the author of the *Feel Good Fast* ebook series, which guides readers through a plant-powered cleanse that will help them lose weight, get back in touch with real food, and feel great. She shares her recipes at www.feelgoodguru.com.

CHEF TAL RONNEN is the author of *The Conscious Cook*. A graduate of the Natural Gourmet Institute, Chef Tal has worked at many major vegan restaurants and prepared the meals for Oprah Winfrey's 21-day vegan cleanse. He conducts master vegetarian workshops at Le Cordon Bleu College campuses nationwide.

CHEF DEL SROUFE of Wellness Forum Foods is known for creating delicious dishes that are not only plant-based, but also low-fat and oil-free. His diverse repertoire guarantees that plant-based diners need never become bored with their food!

ANASTASIA ST. JOHN, based in Ithaca, NY, has over a decade of experience in vegan food preparation. She enjoys creating healthy and delicious fare, to the delight of her friends and family.

JO STEPANIAK, MSEd, the author of *The Ultimate Uncheese Cookbook* and the author or coauthor of fifteen more books, developed the recipes in *Breaking the Food Seduction* by Neal Barnard, MD. Her award-winning column Ask Jo! appears on her Web site, Grassroots Veganism (www.vegsource.com).

DARSHANA THACKER teaches traditional Ayurvedic food preparation at Vapika Spirit in Los Angeles (www.vapikaspirit.com). Her intimate, kitchen-based classes illustrate the simple preparation of well-balanced meals planned according to the season.

BRIAN WENDEL set out to bring the message of plant-based nutrition and health to a broader audience by creating a documentary. He recruited an award-winning production team and spent nearly two years making *Forks Over Knives*, his first feature film.

PERMISSIONS ACKNOWLEDGMENTS

Grateful acknowledgment is made for permission to include (and in some cases to reprint) recipes:

- ► The recipe on page 71 (top) is reproduced by permission of Joey Aucoin.
- ► Recipes on pages 64, 78, 94, 152, 174 (top), 183, and 186 from *Breaking the Food Seduction* by Neal D. Barnard, MD, with recipes from Jo Stepaniak, are copyright © 2003 by the author and reprinted by permission of St. Martin's Press, LLC.
- ► The recipe on page 67 (bottom) is reproduced by permission of Gene Baur.
- ► The recipe on page 160 is reproduced by permission of Yoannah Brown.
- ► Recipes on pages 63, 108 (top), 143, 156–57, 186, and 194 are reproduced by permission of Karen Campbell.
- ► The recipe on page 167 is reproduced by permission of Karen Campbell and LeAnne Campbell Disla.
- ► The recipe on page 107 from *Crazy Sexy Diet* by Kris Carr, copyright © 2011 by Kris Carr, is published by arrangement with the author and skirt!, a division of Globe Pequot Press, Guilford, CT, 06437.
- ► Recipes on pages 155 and 176 are reproduced by permission of Micaela Cook.
- ► Recipes on pages 80, 119 (top), 177, and 193 from the *Whole Plants Cookbook* by LeAnne Campbell Disla, PhD, are reproduced by permission of the author.
- ► Recipes on pages 90, 125, 147, 153, 166, 172, 182, and 184 are reproduced by permission of Ann Esselstyn and Caldwell Esselstyn.
- ► Recipes on pages 105, 108 (bottom), 118 (top), 121, 161–62, and 179 from *Prevent and Reverse Heart Disease* by Caldwell B. Esselstyn Jr., MD, (New York, NY: Avery Books, 2007) are reproduced by permission of the publisher.

► Recipes on pages 65, 119 (bottom), 126–27, 131 (bottom), 168, and 192 from *The Engine 2 Diet* by Rip Esselstyn (New York, NY: Grand Central Books, 2009) are reproduced by permission of the publisher.

► The recipe on page 137 from *Skinny Bitch in the Kitch* by Rory Freedman and Kim Barnouin (Philadelphia, PA: Running Press, 2007) is reproduced by permission of the publisher.

► Recipes on pages 92 and 180 are reproduced by permission of Lewis Freedman and Priscilla Timberlake.

► The recipe on page 91 (bottom) from *Quantum Wellness* by Kathy Freston (New York, NY: Weinstein Books, 2008) is reproduced by permission of the publisher.

► Recipes on pages 76, 85, 109 (top), 120 (top), 150, 171, and 185 from *The Health Promoting Cookbook* by Alan Goldhamer, DC, (Summertown, TN: Book Publishing Company, 1997) are reproduced by permission of the publisher.

► Recipes on pages 66 and 132 are reproduced by permission of Julieanna Hever.

► Recipes on pages 68–69, 88, 95, 102–3, 109 (bottom), 149, 164–65, 174 (bottom), and 187 from *Unprocessed* by Chef AJ with Glen Mercer (CreateSpace, 2011) are reproduced by permission of the author.

► Recipes on pages 71 (bottom), 74, 83, 100, 104, 106, 110, 117 (top), 118 (bottom), 120 (bottom), 123–24, 130–31 (top), 142, 151, 169, 181, and 190 from the "McDougall Newsletters" by John McDougall, MD, and Mary McDougall (Dr. McDougall's Health and Medical Center, www.drmcdougall.com/recipeindex.html) are reproduced by permission of the authors.

► Recipes on pages 89 and 146 are reproduced by permission of Christy Morgan.

► Recipes on pages 112–14 and 158 from *Appetite for Reduction* by Isa Chandra Moskowitz (Cambridge, MA: Da Capo, 2011) are reproduced by permission of the publisher.

► Recipes on pages 82 and 140 are reproduced by permission of Elise Murphy.

► Recipes on pages 79, 96, 111, 117 (bottom), 138–39, 141, 173, 189, and 195–96 are reproduced by permission of Moira Nordholt.

► The recipe on page 170 is reproduced by permission of San'Dera Prude.

► Recipes on pages 75, 91 (top), 101, and 135–36 from *Keep It Simple, Keep It Whole* by Alona Pulde, MD, and Matthew Lederman, MD, (Los Angeles, CA: Exsalus Health & Wellness Center, 2009) are reproduced by permission of the authors.

► Recipes on pages 77, 97, 115, 133–34, 159 and 191 are reproduced by permission of Chef Del Sroufe.

► Recipes on pages 81, 93, 116, 148, and 163 are reproduced by permission of Anastasia St. John.

► Recipes on pages 98–99, 144–45, and 175 are reproduced by permission of Darshana Thacker.

► Recipes on pages 67 (top) and 122 are reproduced by permission of Brian Wendel.

► The recipe on page 154 is reproduced by permission of Anthony Yen.

Acknowledgments

BRIAN WENDEL, executive producer of *Forks Over Knives*

Like the documentary, the *Forks Over Knives* companion book was a collaborative effort of many dedicated people. I would like to acknowledge the work of Gene Stone, our editor, along with that of our contributors, Pam Popper, Micaela Cook, Elise Murphy, and Meghan Murphy; without their time, dedication, and skill, this book simply would not have been possible.

I am grateful to Matthew Lore, the publisher, for taking this project on and for dedicating his time and resources to produce a book that will be lasting. Thank you also to Karen Giangreco, Jack Palmer, and Robby Barbaro for overseeing the important details. And of course, thank you to everyone who generously contributed a recipe. Many of these people are friends and leaders in the healthy plant-based lifestyle movement—a movement that is improving people's lives and making our planet Earth a better place.

GENE STONE, editor

Many, many people contributed to this book. I would like to thank everyone involved with the documentary upon which this book is based, *Forks Over Knives,* especially Brian Wendel, the executive producer, who has poured his life into making this project happen. I am also grateful to all the faces of *Forks Over Knives*—Neal Barnard, Gene Baur, Colin Campbell, Es Esselstyn, Rip Esselstyn, Matt Lederman, Doug Lisle, Terry Mason, John McDougall, Pam Popper, and Alona Pulde—for taking the time from their hectic lives to talk to me. Thanks also to everyone who contributed a recipe or ten!

We were very fortunate to find such a talented publisher willing to take on this project based on a quick conversation and promise to publish almost immediately thereafter: thanks to Matthew Lore and everyone else at The Experiment, to Pauline Neuwirth and her colleagues at Neuwirth and Associates, and to Amy Chamberlain for her sharp copyediting.

Special thanks go to the remarkable Micaela Cook at the T. Colin Campbell Foundation.

Finally, I'd like to thank Miranda Spencer for her wonderful editing, Nick Bromley for his terrific research, and Mark Langley, without whose discerning insights, excellent writing skills, and constant support this book could not have been written.

INDEX

*Page numbers in **bold** indicate a recipe tip.*

ABOUT THE EDITOR

Editor GENE STONE is the author of the international bestseller *The Secrets of People Who Never Get Sick* and the coauthor, with Rip Esselstyn, of *The Engine 2 Diet*. Stone, who has written or ghostwritten more than thirty books and numerous magazine articles, lives in New York and follows a plant-based diet.

ABOUT
FORKS OVER KNIVES

The feature film *Forks Over Knives* examines the profound claim that most, if not all, of the degenerative diseases that afflict us can be controlled, or even reversed, by rejecting animal-based and processed foods. The film traces the personal journeys of Dr. T. Colin Campbell and Dr. Caldwell B. Esselstyn as they uncover more and more evidence for the benefits of a whole-foods, plant-based diet, and features several other experts whose findings corroborate theirs, including Dr. Neal Barnard, Dr. John McDougall, and Dr. Doug Lisle. *Forks Over Knives* also uncovers the history that led to the modern "Western diet"—high in meat, dairy, and processed foods—and presents the challenges and triumphs of several patients with chronic diseases who benefited by switching to a plant-based diet.

Forks Over Knives has garnered attention and support from Dr. Mehmet Oz, Oprah Winfrey, Alicia Silverstone, and John Mackey, CEO of Whole Foods. Roger Ebert concludes, "The bottom line: I am convinced this message is true. A plant-based whole foods diet is healthy. . . . The facts are in."

Forks Over Knives was created by executive producer Brian Wendel, written and directed by Lee Fulkerson, produced by John Corry, and coproduced by Allison Boon. It was filmed over two years at locations all over the United States and in Canada and China. *Forks Over Knives* opened in the United States and Canada in May 2011.